The HEALING RESPONSE

- *Applying The Ten Principles & Laws of Healing*
- *Starter Assessment Tools and Practical Program Tips*
- *Special Sections on Pain, Healing Wounds & Fractures, Irritable Bowel Syndrome, Fatigue & Headaches*

Michael W. Loes, M.D., M.D.(H.)

Disclaimer: This information is presented by an independent medical expert whose sources of information include studies from the world's medical and scientific literature, patient records, and other clinical and anecdotal reports. The material in this book is for informational purposes only and is not intended for the diagnosis or treatment of disease. Please visit a medical health professional for specific diagnosis of any ailments mentioned or discussed in this material.

ISBN 1-893910-18-0
Printed in the United States
Published by Freedom Press
1801 Chart Trail
Topanga, CA 90290
Bulk Orders Available: (800) 959-9797
E-mail: info@freedompressonline.com

ADVANCED PRAISE FOR
the HEALING RESPONSE

"The principles and laws look wonderful—future scientific direction for energy medicine."

> — Harold Bloomfield, M.D., Author, *Hypericum & Depression, Healing Anxiety with Herbs, Finding Peace with Your Past*

"The principles are quite good."

> — C. Norman Shealy, M.D., PH.D. Holos Institute of Health,
> *The Creation Of Health*

"The models you use will appeal to the general reader looking for a way to organize his thoughts about energy medicine. A useful service to patients."

> — Joseph Helms, M.D., Author, *Acupuncture Energetics*
> Founder, UCLA Physician's Program for Medical Acupuncture

"I'm truly impressed with *The Healing Response*. It gets to the core of what a balanced life can be. I believe that if we as physicians really understand and practice these ten laws, we ourselves will have an abundant life and we will help our patients to do the same. The principles and laws will help us move from just being alive into a state where we are abundantly alive. These concepts allow us to look at illness for what it is. It is not our enemy, but a way in which we learn our soul lessons. We need tools with which to work and these ten principles and laws are great tools."

> — Gladys Taylor McGarrey, M.D., M.D.(H)
> Director, Scottsdale Center for Integrative Medicine
> Former Director, Arizona Homeopathic Board
> 2nd President, American Holistic Health Association

"You have underscored the need to look at the healing response in a more holistic and a more scientific way. You have defined what are likely the most important key areas for further research and discussion. Perhaps a couple will eventually be combined, and maybe a few will be added. The thinkers and listeners of the ages will determine this. You have been both practical and philosophical. Both are so important. Your effort is appreciated and should fuel more energy into helping us help people help themselves."

> — Darice Putterman P.T. Diplomate, American
> Academy of Pain Management.
> Director, Valley Therapeutic Services

"*The Healing Response* is quite reasonable and deserves a great deal of thought. I certainly agree in principle and theory with everything you have to say. This is important because unfortunately, we often think of the patient as the problem as opposed to the person who has a problem. Your approach will go a long way to reversing this unfortunate trend, especially in the area of managed care."

> — Thomas J. Romano, M.D., PH.D.
> Diplomate, American Board of Internal Medicine
> Diplomate, American Academy of Pain Management

"As you, and we all in a general sense, attempt to represent the apparent collision between traditional and alternative medical philosophies, I am curious as to what our traditional medical philosophy is. This philosophy is the golden cow that we all seem to be embracing—yet, no such philosophy has ever been clearly outlined for me. If our philosophy is to diagnose disease and treat with prescription drugs, surgery, and radiation therapy, then we need to look further and advance our philosophy and redefine the language we use to express ourselves. I suggest that we use the word medical energetics instead of energetic medicine. This way, the language allows for other types of energetics. I much prefer the term homeodynamics rather than homeostasis. Let us understand that our task is formidable. As we study energetics, we are compelled to attempt measurement of the immeasurable, to define the indefinable and contain that which is not easily caught. This is no small task. In the ancient Greek model of health, there is one disease. It is called 'dys'-'ease,' or in a real sense, 'death of ease.' Manifestations and target organs are myriad. But illness was also thought of as one disease of the holistic being. The ancient Greeks thought of body-mind-spirit as a single thought—i.e., what involved any aspect of the individual person involved the whole. The overriding wish, and the parting word of the Greek physician to his patient was 'Be well l'one (loved one).' Let us train our physicians to love their patients and truly help them in their Quest for Health. Behold, a worthy start."

— Randy Van Nostrand, M.D.
Author, *Quest for Salubrity*
Emergency Medicine Physician,
Website: www.salubrity.com

TABLE OF CONTENTS

ACKNOWLEDGMENTS

A SPECIAL THANKS to staff at the Arizona Pain Institute and Southwest Pain Management Associates: J. Richard Cohen, D.D.S., Steve Fanto, M.D., Barbara Miranda, and Joanne Spangler. Important to note is the research prowess of Neil Cohen, particularly his diligence in searching out resources from the Internet, so crucial in adding the special extra information that seems so elusive when completing a project.

Thank you, David Steinman, M.A., for your mentoring and editorial skills behind this project and encouraging the author to go for the spotlight with a global premier publisher and really get the information out into the airports and WalMarts of America.

To my patients, thank you for allowing me to learn from your problems and letting me into that special relationship of confidence where a treatment plan can be developed and a path to salubrity chosen.

Thank you to my friends and colleagues at Naturally Vitamins, especially Joachim Lehmann, Aftab Ahmed, and John Wolf who gave me the time, encouragement and enthusiasm to keep filling the pen and burning the midnight oil.

To my wife and daughters, a special thank you for being there. It is not easy trying to balance all those mutual responsibilities of life, especially as they relate to family.

I love you all.

—Michael

THE HEALING RESPONSE AND THE TEN PRINCIPLES & LAWS BEHIND IT

THE HEALING RESPONSE is what your body does—its best effort—to get you better when you are threatened with pain or already ill. The *Energetic You* assesses the resources you have and delivers as much healing response as you've got. The resulting healing response is organized and focused on a single goal—getting you healthy again. Your body's ability to accomplish that goal—reclaiming health—depends upon you—the *Energetic You* that goes beyond words and conscious thought—that resides deep within what we call the soul, the spirit, the *anima* and *animus*. I will show you how strong that dependence is and what you can do to assure that your healing response is its most powerful.

There are principles and laws behind *The Healing Response*. Introducing them to you is my purpose. They are to serve as a guide for your healing journey. Are you ready for this educational adventure? Will you allow me to show you how simple it is to make small changes that make a difference? I know I can help.

PRINCIPLE ONE
  Life (The Vital Force) is God-given, however, not necessarily God maintained; free choice exists.
THE LAW
  Build Vital Force and Health Ensues.

PRINCIPLE TWO

Dynamic and Specific Directional Flow of Vital Force Results in Homeostasis (stability in the body).

THE LAW

Enhance Directional Flow and Life Springs.

PRINCIPLE THREE

The Body will make every effort to Preserve Homeodynamics and Avoid Stasis.

THE LAW

Rid Stasis and Healing Happens.

PRINCIPLE FOUR

Diurnal, Lunar and Specific Seasonal Patterns of Energy Flow Exist.

THE LAW

Tune in and Synchronize Your Healing Rhythms.

PRINCIPLE FIVE

Intelligence is in the Cell.

THE LAW

Feed the Cell what it Needs for Health.

PRINCIPLE SIX

The Brain Provides one Level but Not the Only Level of Support to the Cell.

THE LAW

Open all Lines Communicating to the Cell and Vital Exchange Occurs.

PRINCIPLE SEVEN

Our beliefs create a unique biology within us which creates behavior. Equally true is that behavior creates biology which creates beliefs.

THE LAW

Optimize Healthy Beliefs and Behaviors. Expect Speedy Healing.

PRINCIPLE EIGHT
Environment Induces Gene Expression.
THE LAW
Live in a Healthy Environment and Protect against Oxidative Stress.

PRINCIPLE NINE
Toxins exist which assault our structural integrity both internally and externally. Our physical and energetic body must constantly rebuild, shield and actively defend itself.
THE LAW
Enhance, Build and Defend the Fortress to Augment the Healing Response.

PRINCIPLE TEN
A strong connection with God, according to your understanding, positively influences your health and aging. Having spiritual health will slow the rate of aging and dramatically lower incidence of many diseases.
THE LAW
Slow aging and accelerate healing by filling the well of your spiritual reservoir.

The *Ten Principles & Laws of Healing* are offered as a new prism through which to view and treat any injury, sickness, or smoldering illness, whether it be physical, mental, emotional, or spiritual. I want you to attain salubrity—a little-used word with roots in Greek etymology that, translated, means "a state of enviable health."

INTRODUCTION

THE HEALING RESPONSE will rapidly and completely restore normal homeodynamics if you are healthy. If you are not healthy, you must strengthen the healing response, otherwise healing—getting better—will be slow and will not produce the optimal result. In fact, you may become even more sickly. Ultimately, life will cease if your healing response—the *Energetic You*—can't rejuvenate the body when good health begins to slip away.

Learning about the healing response simply requires the practical advice found in this book on how to harness the power of the *Energetic You* for health. It contains practical advice on how to heal quickly and safely. The concept is straightforward, logical and simple to apply. The principles and laws which form the beams and planks of *The Healing Response*, provide both a diagnostic grid and a management formula for understanding your health problems and working systematically to solve them.

Inherent in this information is the fact that your body is not a hodge-podge of multi-colored Playdough® flung together to impact its importance in the world. Life is made up of a unifying energetic harmony of mass (Your Body) and energy (Life Essence). Life is you—the *living, breathing, working person*. A healthy person wakes up feeling charged, focused in purpose, in tune, and connected. If you need help getting back on track, you will find it here.

What we are going to discuss is the "the energetic you." The goal is re-establishing the balance of life forces in you that gives you that ultimate gift: Life lived as you know and dream it can, and should be. Your body's harmony, when healthy, is a confluent balance; it is an equilibrium without division between mind and body. There are no rifts. The spirit in you connects, resonates and touches, going forward in the most uplifting harmony of body, mind, and spirit. Your thoughts, your feelings and your actions are either in concert (Health) or out of tune (dys-ease). If they are not in harmony, you have chaos—serious, malignant disease.

Once chaos begins, it can be like a forest fire on a tinder-dry, windy day. A simple fire extinguisher doesn't exist that can quickly put out flames of chaos. Nor is there a magic potion that will quell the flames. The solution involves mustering the forces—an impregnable fire wall of harmony and spirit. Just like a fire chief, you must assess the situation, take charge and engage the best offensive strategy. When you go boldly forward, undaunted, and singular in purpose, you have a good chance to reclaim salubrity—"the state of enviable health." You rejoice in the relief of quenching the flames of destruction.

Ultimately, your doctor is not your fire department. You cannot lean back and enjoy the results without effort; your doctor, in other words, cannot do for you what you must do for yourself. You are uniquely you. You have the power. You have the responsibility of either choosing to quench the flames with healing water or not. There is information here—important information—that will help you to enhance the healing response. There are real life clinical vignettes from my experience as an internist and algologist (pain management specialist). Here you will see what went wrong and what went right, and how to start and carry through solutions. I will help you to put out the flames of disease and chaos. But you must stay in the chair, listen, digest and ultimately act on this information, and help me to help you pour healing water over the flames.

If you follow the 10 Principles & Laws of Healing that enhance The Healing Response, your life will bear fruit. Here's the door. Put your hand

on the knob. Walk through it. You are not alone. The light is here. I prom-
ise. This is the promised path, the healing path, to salubrity.

—Michael W. Loes, M.D., M.D (H).

Director, Arizona Pain Institute

SALUBRITY: THE SINGULAR GOAL TO HEALTH

We talk a lot about "salubrity," so let's look at this word more carefully. It
is an old English word. It is no longer in the dictionary, though the adjec-
tive—salubrious, meaning a healthy place—lives on in our vocabulary. The
word salubrity is not the kind of word that a street-smart Eliza Doolittle
might utter in the musical *My Fair Lady*. The word is more upper class in
parlance. Perhaps the kind of word—a choice morsel—the English poet
Chaucer might have sprinkled upon an eloquent dialog in *The Canterbury
Tales*. My hope is to introduce to you the concept of salubrity and to teach
the lifestyle behind it. Let's get the word back into common thought and
usage. I have this intent because the concept behind salubrity is rooted in
the Greek tradition of responsible health beliefs and behaviors.

I like to translate salubrity to mean "state of enviable health." This is a
rich idea and worthy goal. But in taking this license, we should explore a
little more of the Greek tradition from where this concept originated; I
want you to know that behind the concept are four pillars felt to be essential to the ancient Greek medical tradition. These pillars underscored that
health is more than the tuning of the body. It has to do with forming a
salubrious web for your life. The web connects you to others and to the
world you live in. The strength of the web results from choices that are
made. The four pillars of salubrity are:

Health: An Integrated State of Being.

Healing: A Process of Integrating the New.

Hospitality: Treating Others as We Would Like to Be Treated.

Responsibility: If not Me, Then Who?

EXPANDING THE LEXICON

There is always a lexicon—a glossary of words that you must know in order to understand and bring together new concepts. There are nearly two hundred words defined in the glossary for this purpose, often briefly discussed and integrated. It might be a good idea to read it first. Assess how many of these words are familiar to you. I don't want to get you distracted or discouraged in your reading. But it is always better to be prepared. Even a few flash cards and other memory aids might be of help to you. Here are a few of the most essential:

Healing: A precise series of actions and reactions directed at restoring the body to homeodynamics.

The Healing Response: The body's best effort to get you well. There are general and specific responses that occur based on the type of problem being encountered and the resources available in your body.

Disease ("Dys Ease"): An alteration in homeodynamics causing a dysfunction of well-being.

Drug: Any substance taken into the body for the purpose of altering physiology to reestablish health. Drugs are given for various reasons, which include fighting infection, and to decrease pain. They may or may not enhance the healing response.

Supplement: Any substance taken into the body presumably to support the body's health.

CONCEPT BEHIND THE HEALING RESPONSE

There are principles and laws behind *The Healing Response*. They build the infrastructure. Each principle makes a general statement followed by an imperative—the law. Each law is the natural advice that flows from the principle. There is then a discussion.

THE CHALLENGE: ASSESSING YOUR HEALTH & RECLAIMING IT

If you don't feel well: If you have early heart disease, your liver is clogging, your sexual function is poor, or your mental attitude is lacking, then changes in your life are going to be necessary to stimulate the healing response. You must be ready to make the move. It is not unlike packing up from a house you loathe or a relationship that is best left behind, and moving on. It takes courage. Perhaps, it takes what you estimate to be your last bit of courage, but you must nevertheless do it. Your reserves are probably better than you think they are. So muster up, gird yourself, and continue. This book can help but I cannot do it for you.

The changes necessary involve an opening of your mind to believe with your heart things that may have seemed superficial in the past. Then, think carefully, and begin connecting your body into wholesome actions. It does not take long, once the commitment has been made, to save your health. When you do this, your biology will change—your physical, emotional, mental and spiritual self will begin to define anew who you really are. Your identity returns or changes for the better.

The central concept of salubrity is that we are social beings who are together on this planet and very dependent on one another. We need mutual nurturing. We are here, not by chance, but by design. The "circle of life" thrives on love and helping one another. Are you up to the challenge? You need to open up. Let the energy flow.

Accept the challenge!

Take on the responsibility!

THE PRINCIPLES & LAWS

Principle & Law One

DEAD BATTERY

THE PRINCIPLE

Life (The Vital Force) is God-Given, however, not necessarily God maintained; free choice exists.

THE LAW

Build Vital Force and Health Ensues.

DISCUSSION

Whether called Energy, Vital Force, Prana, or Kundalini, there is a Life Essence that must be protected. Even the Romans had a name for it—"elan vitale." Perhaps the simple English word "vitality" should be the preferred word. Look around you. You watch people get sick by literally giving their life away. They make poor choices, and just like a car with an oil leak, they let their energy drain away. Also note, that when a person is healthy, they have ample vital force—so much so, that they can boost yours with a hug.

THE EMPHASIS

Make Healthy Choices! Choose to build, support and receive vitality on a constant basis.

Having ample vital force is truly a blessing. How often, as an internist, do I see patients who are tired, weak, dizzy, slow, cold, and in pain? Well, I must tell you that every day I see people like this. Every day. If we could package vital force in a pill or an intravenous liquid, how simple the practice of internal medicine could be! Having ample vital force is like having a full water reservoir. When you feel used up, wouldn't it be nice to simply open up one of the carefully regulated valves and refill the tank?

Vital force is an energy concept. It is not unlike measuring the potential energy in a battery, or how much electricity can be generated by harnessing a waterfall. It is possible to measure vital force. However, this is not calculated because there is no agreement as to which mathematical model would give us the most useful information. An early model of great relevance, which is in fact the foundation of the entire aerobic movement, is the approach taken by Dr. Ken Cooper in dealing with unhealthy air force cadets. These cadets were called "his baby whales." The approach he developed, and which has stood the test of scientific scrutiny, was to measure oxygen utilization with increasing levels of activity. This is the "aerobic capacity," and directly relates to body fitness. As you get into better shape, into better aerobic condition, your aerobic measurement— oxygen/kg/minutes utilization—goes up. When you are overweight, and out of shape, as in military recruits just entering boot camp, you are incapable of doing much of anything and have a very low value. As conditioning occurs, the aerobic capacity increases, and so does the ability to do the many requirements of being a successful soldier. Any of Dr. Cooper's books are useful reading to review this concept, which in effect measures vitality. (*Aerobics, The New Aerobics, Aerobics for Women, The Aerobic Way*)

Another approach, dear to the heart of bariatricians (doctors specializing in weight control), is to measure the basal metabolic rate. This can be done by measuring early morning temperatures and correlating them with weight and pulse. Traditionally, this test was done to measure thyroid function before testing blood levels became fashionable. An exercise advocate for this type of approach is Covert Bailey, who believes that health—and ability to maintain your weight—has to do with the "size of your engine" which is determined by percent body fat, and basal metabolic rate.

Psychologists will use the concept of stress reserve. Whether a life stress scale is done or a rat is put through the maze, information can be obtained that will relate to disease development and vitality of the subject. I am certain—my intuition tells me—that people with ample stress reserve could be shown to live longer. We just haven't done the study yet but people who handle stress well, who have a mission in life, and who understand that the sprint to the finish comes *after* the marathon has been run, know that the key to longevity has something to do with stress. They learn to handle it. It is vitally related to their vitality.

Lab chemists look at cells all day and they might have looked at yours or mine at one time or another. Cells can be stimulated with various triggers of varying strengths. Cells can be made to run, hide, or kill. Scientists can measure how an individual's cells handle dangerous bacteria, poisons, or other threats to life. A healthy cell has vitality; it can be measured. It is like measuring the immune system of each member of your army.

Our brains have power. The power can be asserted symmetrically or asymmetrically. Measuring power coherence of the right and left brain can be done. This field of neurological assessment is called quantitative electroencephalopathy. Assessments can also be made metabolically and this area of neurological assessment is called functional MRI (Magnetic Resonance Imaging). A healthy strong electrical and metabolic picture surely relates to good health and longevity.

Many areas of medicine have their energetic assessment techniques. The acupuncturists have theirs, as do the homeopaths, the chiropractors, and the kinesiologists. They are measuring vital force and improving it.

Assessing vital force—the abundance or lack of it—is without a doubt, a very useful medical tool. We need to take the effort to understand the physiology, chemistry and physics behind it. We need to take a step further and begin to clinically use it for the benefit of ourselves. Doing this will help us reclaim salubrity.

Let me tell you about Mark. He lost his vital force and expended his vital reserves.

CLINICAL VIGNETTE #1

Mark has systemic Lyme Disease. This illness is acquired from a North American tick, which then triggers an abnormal immune response. When caught early, there are antibiotics that kill the organism and arrest the disease. Mark was unfortunate. Even though he was a dentist, and quickly recognized that there was something wrong, he either didn't get started on therapy soon enough, or was just one of those people who didn't respond. He is tired all the time but can't sleep. He is in pain all the time, but even strong narcotic drugs (opioids) do not seem to help his pain much. He describes a "mental fog" —he just can't think, and coffee doesn't help. Even strong prescription stimulants just don't seem to work. Mark brings with him the long list of drugs he has tried. The list is over a hundred. Not only has Mark lost his health, but his wife now sleeps in a different bedroom because he is so moody and unpredictable. His 16-year-old son has moved out, and his 14-year-old daughter doesn't seem to want to talk to him anymore. He is drained and the drainage is more than just physical. His mind is failing. His mood is overwhelmingly depressed and his spirit has collapsed.

Mark has now decided to reduce his medications. He has quit taking sleep aids, caffeine, and tranquilizers. He is taking Ester C®, four grams per day, and slow release magnesium. He is walking every day with his wife.

Mark is not well. He probably will never again regain Salubrity. But God performs miracles: We just don't know if he has one in store for Mark. The goal is to shift the sails of Mark's ship. Hopefully, he can then pick up a little healing wind. If that happens, perhaps he can pick up some healing response and augment it. Hopefully, he can then reset his course and reclaim salubrity.

As an internist, I don't have intravenous vital force. I wish I did. Mark needs to fill his tank or have it filled for him. I think he can do it. Let me tell you how...

THE METAPHOR

Having problems with absence of vitality is like having a dead battery. You must find a way to charge it up. There are ways of conserving energy and ways of making sure it sparks up more effectively. Certain cellular energizers may be worthwhile considering such as coenzyme Q_{10}, NADH, and inulin. Oxygen is, of course, a cell energizer. Make sure your air is clean and plentiful. Walk in the forest where the air is charged with vital force.

Principle & Law Two
BLOCKED HIGHWAY

THE PRINCIPLE

Dynamic and Specific Directional Flow of Vital Force Results in Homeodynamics.

THE LAW

Enhance Directional Flow and Life Springs.

ENHANCEMENT

Preserving natural and adequate movement of Vital Force is essential. Moving our bodies assures we get enough blood and oxygen. Just as blood flows in one direction, so does energy. Study the deep and superficial pathways of Traditional Chinese Medicine.

THE EMPHASIS

Get Directional Energetic Therapy—massage, acupuncture, acupressure.

DISCUSSION

The concepts of Traditional Chinese Medicine (TCM) are very clear about the directional flow of chi (pronounced 'chee'). There are designated paths, both on a superficial level ("wei chi") and a deeper level (meridian flow, and eu-mo channels). There may be reservoir points where energy can build up, but there is not backward flow. Examples are the kidneys, which are so important to our energy reserves and flow.

It should be underscored that the basis of confusion in discussing a concept is often related to a poor understanding of defining terms. You can choose to define a "negative energy" and then this principle and law would not be true. We are talking about the energy behind The Healing Response. Healing energy flows in one direction—the direction necessary to heal.

Measuring the Direction Flow

You can measure it. There are several oriental techniques, one of which is called "akabani." You simply count the time it takes for chi to arrive at a specific acupuncture point called a "ting point." Meridian flow has been measured (see the milestone text which defines American acupuncture by Joseph Helms, *Acupuncture Energetics*, and the multiple works of Dr. Francois Mussat, who was the primary lecturer for over a decade in the UCLA courses on acupuncture energetics). Critics would like you to believe that "chi" is unseen and immeasurable spiritualism. This is just not true. We know the force of the electrical charge generated by an acupuncture needle. We know how fast the chi moves in the meridian channels (three to five centimeters per second). We even know which endorphins are stimulated by which frequencies known as electrical acupuncture. We also know about directional force fields. Of particular importance is the cornerstone work of Dr. Robert Becker, an orthopedic surgeon who studied salamanders and limb regeneration. A certain directional force field had to be applied and the limb would regenerate. If the direction was changed, the limb would not regenerate. Dr. Becker is a popular speaker and his work is summarized in his books, *The Body Electric* and *Cross Currents*. His enthusiasm and mentoring of other investigators has resulted in a burgeoning of information relating to healing micro-currents.

CLINICAL VIGNETTE #2

Shannon is a 29-year-old Caucasian female who has been experiencing lower pelvic pain for 3 years. She has been told that she has endometriosis, and has had two surgeries to remove "benign" masses, as her gynecologist calls them. She is told that there is no medication for this, although hormone suppression has been suggested. On further questioning, she has a lot of bloating, gas, and constipation. She asks her gynecologist about acupuncture, but he politely scoffs at the question.

Quite unexpectedly, her gynecologist calls and says that he does know of a physician who was trained through the UCLA extension program in acupuncture. She schedules an appointment and is surprised that the office looks like that of a internal medicine physician: no voodoo dolls, mysterious music or scents. Even the artwork looks conservative. The evaluation involves a rather long taking of the pulse, a careful look at the tongue, and then a search for tender points. She is treated bilaterally with only six needles on the first visit: medial calf (Sp6), lateral and inferior kneecap (St36), and outer ankle (Bl60). Some very mild hand stimulation (twisting) of tiny needles is performed for twenty minutes. Even after the first treatment, Shannon sleeps better. After six treatments, her pelvic pain is gone and she feels the bloating and congestion in her pelvis is better. She feels more like "a normal woman" again.

CLINICAL VIGNETTE #3

Lisa Montefiore is 29 years old and was healthy until a year and a half ago. She was involved in a car accident where she severely twisted her back and neck. She has been living in constant pain, unable to even sit on a sofa, lay on her stomach, or stand longer than five minutes. She thought her days as an active horsewoman were over. The pain pills her doctors prescribed left her dizzy, nauseated, and reeling with headaches. A physical therapist's traction treatments only increased the throbbing she constantly had in her neck.

Lisa cringed when her family doctor and then her daughter's tai chi instructor suggested acupuncture. Having needles stuck into her body seemed to her the worst kind of torture. The neurologist, the orthopedist, and the pain specialist she consulted all dismissed the idea. But Lisa, worn down by relentless pain, was desperate and ready to try anything.

Lisa was skeptical when she went to her first appointment with Dr. Bradley Williams, a family doctor in Phoenix who has been integrating acupuncture into his practice for the past fifteen years. After a nurse took Lisa's blood pressure, Dr. Williams came in and began to ask detailed questions. Where did she hurt most? What aggravated her discomfort? How far could she bend over? How would she rate her pain on a scale of one to ten? They talked for a few more minutes, then Dr. Williams studied her pulse and tongue, two diagnostic keys in Traditional Chinese Medicine.

Finally, it was time for the needles. Lisa stiffened in anticipation as Dr. Williams pressed the skin on the back of her neck to find the right point. She squeezed her eyes tight, waiting for the flash of pain. But when the needle went in, she felt less than a pinprick, a sensation that lasted only an instant. As he inserted more needles in her back, stomach, and feet—some as little as one-sixteenth of an inch deep, others as much as two inches—she began to feel calm, even sleepy.

Half an hour later, Dr. Williams came back to remove the needles, and asked Lisa how she was feeling. "My pain was down from about a ten to a four or a five," she said. During the next few months, she had nine more treatments, and left all but one of them feeling better (she recalled cramping after one session when electrostimulation was used).

More than two-and-a-half years after the car accident, Lisa still isn't completely healed. She feels some pressure in her back when her horse moves into a trot. But at least she is riding again. If she spends a long afternoon sitting at one of her daughter's horse shows, she is sore for a couple of days. But acupuncture has done what the drugs and physical therapy couldn't. It has restored her life. "I figure my back will never be like it was before," she says. "But I'm not in pain. It's more like an ache or discomfort. I can pick up a bag of groceries or walk my horse now."

Last fall, shortly after telling her State Farms claims adjuster how much better she felt, Lisa received a surprise in the mail: a check for $1,450—the full cost of the treatment. Just a few months before, the insurer had said it wouldn't pay *a penny. Apparently Lisa was very persuasive, or State Farm is coming around to the obvious conclusion: That acupuncture works. As the Smith-Barney ad talks about "one investor at a time," perhaps investing in "one life at a time" could and should become a good investment for insurers as well.*

Today, we are seeing a "coming around" to the idea and acceptance of some, but not all, of the alternative, now called "integrative," therapies. It's about time.

Acupuncture, acupressure, and craniosacral therapy are all examples of strategic healing techniques that focus on moving healing energy in the direction it is meant to move. Their availability is now widespread. Even at the Mayo Clinic in Scottsdale, an acupuncturist has been added. Less than five years ago, when I was a member of the faculty there, such a thought would have been summarily rejected.

THE METAPHOR

When you have a blocked energy flow pattern, it is like driving, or attempting to drive on a highway where there is an obstruction, as in a motor vehicle accident where a truck is rolled in your path. You must unblock the highway to reach your destination.

Principle & Law Three

DEAD SEA/STAGNANT POND

THE PRINCIPLE

The Body will make every effort to Preserve Homeodynamics and Avoid Stasis.

THE LAW

Rid Stasis and Healing Happens.

ENHANCEMENT

Stasis is a cardinal concept for explaining the etiology of illnesses. If you clog the system, swelling and inflammation occur. There is immediate acute inflammation: redness, swelling, heat, and pain. There is fever, as the body heats up to rid the stasis. If the blockage is not cleared, fibrosis and sclerosis develop which leads to coldness, disuse and atrophy. Chronic pain is too often the consequence.

DISCUSSION

What does this term "homeodynamics" mean? It means having a perfectly tuned Steinway piano, with a master pianist at the keyboard. The intelligent and talented pianist performs. He (or she) not only plays the notes, but knows when he hits the right notes. He then augments the melody and the result is a symphony. We cherish the experience.

Well, if you're not into music, let me give another example: Homeodynamics is having just the right Harley Davidson. The "hog" that feels like the perfect fit for your pelvis that vibrates with the signature roar of the engine. The ultimate magic is in the ride, not just the feeling of the straddle. The intelligent rider who knows the bike like his own soul is crucially important to the orgasmic thrill of the journey. Here is harmony. Here is the perfect combination of structure and life force. Homeostasis—yes, but also homeodynamics.

Let's look at a few more symptoms of stasis or blockages, especially as they relate to the holistic you—the physical, the emotional, the mental and the spiritual.

PHYSICAL STASIS

- Do you find yourself swelling later in the day? Are your ankles puffy and is there congestion in your legs? This is stasis—likely kidney stasis that may also involve the liver and heart.
- Do you find rings, and a slight darkening under your eyes? This is also a sign of kidney congestion.
- Your urine is foul smelling, and a little brown in coloration. This is stasis in the liver.
- You are short of breath, and feel congested in the lungs. This is a slowing or blockage of energy flow in the lungs—pulmonary stasis.
- You are tired, and your blood pressure is low. This is heart stasis.
- Your joints are hot. This is acute inflammation, and there is clogging of inflammatory material in the area of pain—musculoskeletal stasis.
- Your joints are cold. This is chronic inflammation characteristic of fibrosis, sclerosis, and degeneration—systemic stasis.

EMOTIONAL STASIS

- Do you have a bitter root pulling you down?
- Are you jealous, or burning with envy regarding a lost love, or an occupational goal?

- Are you just running away with tears? You just can't dry them up?
- Are you angry all the time and apt to let loose with obscenities or unkind, demeaning words?

MENTAL STASIS

- Are you having problems with forgetfulness? You just don't have the energy—or brain—to remember? The causes can be multiple, likely not enough sleep or an imbalance of intruding thoughts and emotional blockages.
- Are you having problems speaking clearly? Are the words and thoughts coming out jumbled? Are your thoughts disordered and your thinking hazy?
- Are you an insomniac? You just can't sleep because your mind is filled to the brim with worried thoughts?
- Are you obsessed with a pain problem? You feel that you are telescoping right to a painful area of your body—your abdomen, your pelvis? Your mind is stuck—there is nothing else you can think about. You must move beyond this energetically. This is mental stasis.
- Have you ever been unable to make up your mind about something? You feel locked, just like the magician wrapped in knotted ropes and dropped in the swimming pool. Have you felt that way?
- Have you made a decision and then wanted to "take it back?" Maybe you bought something. The credit card bill has not even come yet. It is still new, still in the bag. You could take it back. You made the decision to buy it and now you want to undo the decision?
- What about the first time you gave your love away. Do you wish you could undo that decision?
- You just sent your child off to college, or perhaps on a mission trip? Perhaps to a place that is not that safe—like Guatemala? Is your brain bruised by a crisis?

SPIRITUAL STASIS

- Are you holding a grudge?
- Do you refuse to forgive?
- Do you suffer guilt and you just can't get rid of it?
- Are you lost and nameless? You just don't fit in anywhere?
- Do you sense your worth somewhere between a penny and less than zero?

The solution to stasis will always involve "movement," whether movement of your body, or movement of the heart or mind.

There are ways of "unblocking." Some of these are physical, such as getting more exercise, doing things that increase your oxygen, for example supplementing your diet with coenzyme Q_{10} or *Gingko biloba*. There are ways of getting through an emotional block—such as hypnosis or Traeger rebirthing techniques. Mentally, getting a friend that listens and encourages will help to break a block. Going to church or confession, or involvement in a ministry, will break open your spiritual life. But you have to move.

THE METAPHOR

Having a problem with stasis is like examining the Dead Sea and trying to find a solution. Just over the hill is the Sea of Galilee and it is teeming with fish, plants, and other wildlife. You discover that the only difference in these two bodies of water is that the Dead Sea has no outlet, only an inlet. The Sea of Galilee has an inlet and an outlet. Take a trip to Israel. Find out for yourself.

Principle & Law Four
WRECKED RHYTHM

THE PRINCIPLE

Biological Rhythms are Essential to Optimal Health. These can be diurnal, lunar or seasonal. They may even be characteristic of certain stages of our unique life.

THE LAW

Tune in, Synchronize, and Reset Temporal Rhythms.

ENHANCEMENT

Just as there are times and seasons for illness, so also are there optimal times to heal. Be informed and aware of temporal cycles, whether it is the Horare Clock of Chi Movement, Monthly Hormonal Cycles, Seasonal Illnesses, or Years for Bounty or Calamity. We know timing is important for pregnancy, allergy shots, and even chemotherapy. We know that there are times when depression is more severe and seasons where the mind is more open to positive thoughts.

EMPHASIS

Know the Time and Tune into Healing Rhythms.
Choose the Optimal Time and Season to Heal.

DISCUSSION

Perhaps Jewish history is the best place to start a discussion about "Choosing the Right Time." From the times of Abraham to Christ's Apostles, there are references about choosing the right or wrong time. The Talmud—book of Jewish Law—devotes up to a third of its precepts and precautions around time—the right and proper time. There is a time to plant and a time to harvest. There is a time to let the field be barren (every seven years). There are years of scarcity and those of plenty. There are times to be wed and to romance. There are specified times to care for the sick. There are times to heal and times not to be healed. There are also times to eat, to celebrate with food, and to fast—abstaining from food.

The study of daily biological rhythms is called the study of circadian rhythms. There are also infradian rhythms. These are cycles that are more than a day, like menstrual cycles, or cycles of the white blood corpuscles. There are also shorter rhythms called ultradian rhythms—less than a day. These are the cycles of adrenalin, of testosterone and in Traditional Chinese Medicine, the movement of chi through an organ system. It is known that the peak activity of stomach chi is between 7:00 a.m. and 9:00 a.m. and for sexual energy it is between 9:00 p.m. and 11:00 p.m. Does this surprise you? Time is vitally important. Our biological system is intricately tied to and dependent on having enough time to do what needs to be done. This area of investigation is called chronobiology—the study of time as it relates to biology. Some of the pioneering work was done by Dr. Charles F. Ehret and reviewed in his book *Overcoming Jet Lag*. More recently, much of this research has been reviewed in *The Circadian Prescription*, a book by Sidney MacDonald Barker, recipient of the 1999 Linus Pauling award.

CLINICAL VIGNETTE #4

John, a 37-year-old Roman Catholic, kept seeking a life—a life of harmony, a life pleasing to Jesus Christ. In his teens, he dated, and in fact had a steady girl-friend that now he thinks he should have married; but to him, the "timing wasn't right." In his twenties, he got involved in Catholic charity work, which he felt was pleasing to God, but he wasn't really happy. He became discouraged when he found that the charity was managed more like a business than a ministry, and many of his co-workers didn't share his love and compassionate feelings; they just wanted to get the job done and go home. John met another girl in the ministry and, for a short time, he thought that they might get married. The time went by quickly. It never happened.

John became very depressed. He was trapped in life evaluation and not living. He found that his old friends had moved on and the significant relationships he'd had, passed him by. Now, they were just memories, old memories—painful ones. John began to eat less and less and became malnourished. He was treated with anti-depressants, but these did not seem to work.

At the suggestion of his therapist, John joined a group for eating disorders. He felt some bonding in that depression was a commonly shared experience within the group.

John is now nearing forty. He is looking for a new identity. He knows that the time is soon—perhaps in the spring, he will reach out and do something that is just slightly out of his comfort zone. He is being encouraged to put time in perspective, and notice a new beginning. It is time. It is always time to recognize our rhythms, be they short, long or for a lifetime. Act within your rhythms. Keep the symphony in your head or the feeling of the Harley hog.

John's case is included here to alarm you. Perhaps you too are bogged down in self-reflection and uncertainty, and not willing to pick the time and move into a forward wave toward better health.

CLINICAL VIGNETTE #5

Jasper is a 20-year-old college student who doesn't sleep well. He admits that he is a little "driven," wanting to take all of the required courses, and then some—to get ahead and perhaps graduate a semester early. To top it off, finances are tight and a part-time job has become necessary. To be flexible, he takes a busing job at an all-night restaurant, and tries to work two to three eight-hour shifts per week.

Armed with a young healthy body, an appreciation for caffeine, and power bars he does okay for a few weeks into the semester. By the time midterms are upon him, the stress is building to a breaking point. Sleep is getting poorer, ability to concentrate is lessening, and the homework assignments are becoming overdue.

He begins experiencing classic stress responses: Fast heart rate, sweating, urinary urgency, and he begins having some word-finding problems. He feels a little tight in the chest, is clenching his jaw, and having some early morning headaches. He senses that a little paranoia is building and he gets tense when the phone rings. His bowels are irregular and his appetite seems forced and inconsistent.

Much like a quarterback in the quicksand, he gropes for help. His parents' help is sought, and some brakes are applied to the situation. The part-time job is immediately stopped. The principles of circadian eating are emphasized: protein in the morning, a little extra carbohydrates in the evening, and avoidance of all caffeine-containing beverages after four p.m. Small lunches are appropriately scheduled. Some restraints on the social life are clamped into place. A set bedtime is agreed upon, and Jasper is to use three to six milligrams of melatonin as a sleep aid for the first couple of weeks.

It doesn't take long before Jasper feels a whole lot better. What was needed was the redevelopment of a reverence for the time factor. It is too easy to negate it out of the daily calendar, and foolishly hope that everything is going to fall into place.

Sometimes it takes a lot of lessons to learn a lesson. Sometimes these lessons are learned too late—when chronic disease and unhealthy life styles have already been firmly set. Respect time and it will be good to you. Hopefully, Jasper is learning this lesson soon enough to reclaim salubrity.

We must pay attention to time. It is no surprise that there is a time for finding a lifetime marital companion, as in John's case. If the time passes, it cannot easily be reclaimed. The clock ticks on. How often do we not tune in? Do you make excuses for not acting? We need to notice, to tune in and get onto the wave of sustaining and healing time.

THE METAPHOR

A discordant song or an out-of-tune instrument is familiar enough to all of us with children in music lessons. Do we just sit back and listen uncomfortably or do we try to make the problem go away? With proper instruction, our children will become musicians. An instrument can be restrung and rhythm taught once we get in tune with our body. Awareness is the key here and this must be followed by corrective action. Solve the wrecked rhythm problem. Your life may depend on it.

Principle & Law Five
SQUAWKING CELL

PRINCIPLE
Intelligence is in the Cell.

LAW
Feed the Cell what it Needs for Health.

ENHANCEMENT
The human body responds automatically to most conditions. It does so at a cellular level. We are used to talking about reflexes and the autonomic nervous system (i.e., the system of nerves and nerve cells in the blood vessels, heart, smooth muscles, viscera and glands that controls their involuntary functions). But we usually think of our brain as the central headquarters for our nervous system. Why is it so difficult to admit that very likely our brain has been the recipient of too much credit? Perhaps, we need to pay more attention to our "gut reaction," for it is within our gastrointestinal tract that a cellular surveillance system exists that is a lot more independent than we think. When a problem is detected, the system sends out a corrective action. The action may be cellular, hormonal, humoral, or neural. The emphasis is that a healing response occurs and does so without our brains ever being aware of the action taken.

To understand this phenomenon, a more open model is required. An understanding of receptors is just not broad enough to answer the necessary questions. We need to understand the nature of the challenges and the specifics of the resulting healing response. Energetic science has advanced sufficiently to seriously undertake this task. The problem has been that it is still not on the medical school agenda. Medical physicians seldom advance their understanding of science once they enter practice. They may learn about new drugs or a new procedure, but to undertake a new way of thinking about cellular intelligence is perhaps being left for the next generation of physicians. If that is the case, at least this is a starting point that must be underscored.

We know that when that surveillance system is defective, when our shields are down, or the necessary minerals, vitamins, nutrients, and phytochemicals or cellular protectors are deficient or are not present, disease occurs.

THE EMPHASIS
Feed the Cell what it needs for health!

DISCUSSION
Have you ever watched an amoeba? (Well, probably not, unless you were a biology major or medical school student.) This unicellular protozoan has been the object of biology students since at least the advent of the microscope. Here is a one-cell mass of cytoplasma that takes in food and sends out waste; it does so quite intelligently. Messages go in and out through the cell membrane. The amoeba can respond to danger—move away from it even though it does not have a brain. For all practical purposes, it can "think." Hmm. How far away are we really from an amoeba? In some ways, not far at all.

In *The Second Brain*, author Michael Gershon, M.D., a prominent anatomist and gastroenterologist at Columbia University, devotes a discussion to research involving the autonomy and intelligence of the enteric nervous system, which is, according to Dr. Gershon and others, the second brain. Especially important are the cells lining the intestine—"M" cells in the Peyer's Patches (lymphoid organs in the tissue of the gut). Dr. Gershon details how the cerebral cortex does not control the gut; it is, more or less, independent. He points out that you cannot live without your gut. He reviews experiments wherein animals were decorticated (brains removed), then fed food either directly into the stomach by a tube, or even down the esophagus. They were able to digest the food. The implication is that when it comes to basic survival, you are perhaps better off with your gut than with your cerebral cortex. So perhaps you should listen more to "your gut reaction" and less to your brain or your articulate colleagues who may also not be in touch with their guts!

One might think that understanding what the cell needs is complicated. Rarely is this the case. Most of the time we know. Our "gut reaction" is more often than not that on which we should rely.

PRACTICAL ADVICE: CELL NEEDS

○ Cells do not like to be dehydrated. Give them plenty of uncontaminated water and they will thrive.

○ Cells power up with minerals because of their battery effect. Give them the necessary minerals.

○ Cells do not like to be hypoxic. Oxygen must be abundant, and not full of sulfites, particulates, or carbon monoxide. Cells do not like the vasoconstrictive effect of the nicotine in cigarettes or the tars that wreck air membrane transport in the lungs.

○ Cells do not like alcohol. Alcohol, in any significant quantity, will anesthetize them, making them cold and sluggish. Yes, there is a little trans-resveratrol in alcohol, especially red wine. Perhaps, the antioxidant effect of this compound will lessen the risk of heart disease in a few people who are predisposed. But seriously, this is unlikely and you can get plenty of this beneficial antioxidant effect by taking some supplemental grapeseed extract.

METAPHOR

We have an integrated intelligence that coordinates the combined information from the brain and other parts of our body. The perception and relay of information occurs primarily at a cellular level—and some would argue even at the molecular level where transcription RNA is regulated. We must pay attention to the small components, because where there is a hungry cell, a weak cell, or a poisoned cell, disease begins. We need to ensure that it does not. If your cells are squawking, listen. They have an important message.

Take a Healing Interlude

COOL, COOL, WATER

" Don't treat thirst with medications. Medications are palliatives. They are not designed to cure the degenerative diseases of the human body."
> — Fereydoon Batmanghelidj, M.D. *Your Body's Many Cries For Water* (Global Health Solutions 1997)

CELLS NEED TO HAVE THEIR ESSENTIALS MET. So obvious, but so neglected, is the body's need for water, the solvent that comprises 75 percent of our body weight. In a culture so driven by the bottling industries, most notably Coca Cola and Pepsi, we have been duped to believe that specialized liquids (soda pop) can somehow be a salubrious substitute for water. We have come to believe that you can meet a thirst with liquids, instead of water. This is so far from the truth an alarm must be sounded. Dehydration may be the cause or perpetuator of many chronic illnesses. Without adequate water there is mineral buildup, causing kidney stones, cholesterol plaque that contributes to heart disease, bacterial overcrowding in the intestine causing toxic waste accumulation, and productions of endotoxins. Avoiding such toxicity build-up and assuring a flowing vital stream are key defenses against conditions such as asthma, angina, cirrhosis, kidney disease, ulcers, even constipation.

Dehydration is a cause of accelerated aging and chronic disease. When you are twenty years old, most of your body water is inside the cells—about 60 percent. This percentage declines with age, being about 50 percent at age fifty, reducing to 40 percent by age eighty. Why this happens is more likely related to choice than to anything specific that happens to the cells. The cell numbers do not change significantly. It is likely that there are changes in cell membranes, most aptly described as "hardening," which may make water less mobile through the membranes—but none of this is known for sure. It is an observation worth recalling especially when you are choosing what and how much to drink at your next meal.

HOW MUCH WATER DO WE NEED?

Water need, like other nutrients, is somewhat variable dependent on climate, activity requirements, and specialized needs. As a general rule, you should consume daily about half as much water in ounces as body weight in pounds.

Example: If you weigh 160 pounds, you need about 80 ounces of water on a daily basis as a minimum. If you want to calculate that in six-pack terms, that would be a little more than a six-pack—6.67 of the familiar sized Coke cans.

What are the properties of water, besides its solvent properties, that makes it so crucial to our health?

○ Water-dependent hydrolysis is one of the most common chemical reactions in the body. This reaction cleaves much of the food that we eat into smaller components, so that the smaller particles can be absorbed and used by the body to both sustain and grow.
○ Water produces hydroelectric energy (voltage). This voltage helps to maintain the battery power in the conversion of adenosine triphosphate to guanidine triphosphate (GTP), the vital phosphorus energy bonds that are so crucial to get up and go.
○ Water is part of our structure and is intricately woven into the adhesion material in muscles, collagen, and even bones.

○ Waterways transport messenger molecules, especially nerve messages.
○ Water is the preferred environment for enzymes as they identify and either build or remove vital infrastructure for our bodies.

We are in trouble. Our health is being daily challenged, often by drugs that are counterproductive to bodily drought management. Many of the drugs that are aimed at making us feel transiently better, such as those that effect swelling in the ankles (diuretics), lower blood pressure (renin blocking agents), or reduce inflammation (NSAIDs), dry us out, increasing the risk of our cells sticking together, weakening us and giving us the blahs. Drugs that lower cholesterol, lower glucose, and lower uric acid may make the numbers look better but are messing with our primary and subordinate systems of water management. Antibiotics irritate the gastrointestinal tract, change the friendly microflora, reduce the ability of the intestine to absorb water, and in doing so make water less available to our healing pathways.

Not only do these drugs cause confusing side effects (dry mouth, nausea), they often directly affect the spigot flow of vital homeostatic mechanisms, often overloading or causing unusual stress on the cardiovascular, renal or hepatic systems.

Sometimes, but less often than is traditionally done, strong, potent pharmacology is necessary to literally save a patient from the grips of death, as in septic shock, or pulmonary edema. When an emergency occurs, emergency treatment is required. But this is usually not the case, and conservative care and the utmost respect for our water management system is necessary and deserved.

When drying is allowed to continue unchecked, many vital systems begin to either stick or shut down entirely. One such vital system is the pulmonary system where large quantities of mucus (which is itself 98 percent water) is voluminously produced when there are allergies or infection. When mucus is inadequate, the infection goes deep, which means that it invades the actual lung tissue, causing pneumonia. Water can protect from these developments. When mucus does not allow the toxins to be excreted, they can pass into the cells and cause cellular changes. Smoking accelerates the dryness and impedes mucus production. The cumulative result of long-term smoking can be the development of lung cancer. Its appearance does not surprise those familiar with optimal water management.

When water is unavailable to joints, a similar scenario occurs. Water makes up to 95 percent of the viscosity of joint synovial fluid. When it becomes thick, joints stick, creak, and sometimes "snap, crackle and pop." This makes them prone to injury and the development of chronic inflammation known as arthritis (i.e., "fire in the joints"). The pharmaceutical industry has gone so far as to develop artificial joint fluids, which will temporarily help to improve the viscosity of the joint fluid, but these are not the answer. Hydration—water—is.

Does the brain need water? *Absolutely*—even more than other tissues. The brain is 85 percent water and has complex electrical networks that power the chemistry of messaging. It should not surprise you that depression is associated with dehydration and that, when exposed to stress, cortisol and adrenalin are produced, causing vasoconstriction and dehydration. When one does not sleep because of anxiety and stress, there is further dysfunction of the water management system, and more and more disruptions of normal body biodynamic mechanisms.

We are a beverage-consuming society. Not only do most beverages not help hydration, they can make things worse. Many actually contain diuretics. A beer drinker does not need a lot of convincing that alcohol causes a diuretic action. This can be so powerful and socially awkward that many beer drinkers put salt in their beer to delay its onset. The same can be said of coffee, tea and the various colas on the market today, diet or otherwise. If you are drinking beverages instead of water, you will run an increased risk of dehydration, and the multiple chronic diseases that can result from water deficiency.

Save money and save your health. Reclaim your salubrity. Drink a glass of cool, cool water. And another.

Principle & Law Six

TOWER OF BABEL

THE PRINCIPLE
The Brain Provides One Level, but Not the Only Level of Support to the Cell.

THE LAW
Open All Lines Communicating to the Cell—Vital Exchange Occurs.

ENHANCEMENT
Communication is a complex exchange of information. It must be given and received. Making this exchange effective is the key to a mutual understanding of what needs to happen. Knowledge of how cells communicate is not totally obscure. The wider gap is accepting that our brain is not the speaker. Neuropeptides and hormones are doing the communicating and most of it is automatic. The language bits are relayed either by the blood stream (humoral) or by energetic pathways such as neural connectors. Receptors receive and process these messengers. This communication is more than physical. Body language or a "gut reaction" incites and excites molecules. Verbal communication can open cellular channels. Positive emotional exchanges can powerfully enhance healing. Try forgiveness. It is surely a channel-opener.

THE EMPHASIS

Learn the Language of the Cell! Understand Messenger Physiology!

DISCUSSION

Cells speak to one another through messengers going back and forth from cell to cell through blood, via tissues and even the cytoplasm of the cells—everywhere. The infrastructure of the messaging system is complicated but understood fairly well on a physiological and even biochemical basis. Some messengers must go through membranes to deliver the data. Here is where lipophilic and hydrophilic factors become important. Other messengers activate intermediary signaling stations on the outer membrane.

Some of these messengers have familiar names such as histamine, adrenalin, endorphins, and serotonin. Others are less well known: glutamate, aspartate, and substance P, which are peripheral neurotransmitters. In the brain, there is dopamine, gamma-aminobutyric acid (GABA), noradrenalin, and serotonin, of which there are many subtypes. There are endorphins: beta-endorphin, enkephalin, and dynorphins. There are also prostaglandins and many other pro-inflammatory mediators, especially PGE-2. The work of Dr. Candace Peart in *Molecules of Emotion* is seminal.

There are anti-inflammatory tissue enzymes. One such system is known as the cyclo-oxygenase enzyme system known respectively as COX-1 and COX-2. Selectively inhibiting COX-2 is being heralded as one of the most important molecular advances of the decade, because a way has been found to ward off inflammation without incurring serious gastrointestinal toxicity when COX-1 is unintentionally inhibited. The success of the new arthritis drugs celecoxib (Celebrex) and rofecoxib (Vioxx) attest to this sizzling level of interest.

There are vascular control messengers: prostacyclin A-2 (vasodilation and smooth muscle relaxation), thromboxane A-2 (vasoconstriction and platelet aggregation), bradykinin, thromboxane, and kallikrein (inflammation).

There are eicosanoids, interleukins, and genetic enzymes that regulate carrier molecules such as alpha globulin—fast and slow form. There is a cascade of complements that help inactivate immune complexes.

Let's open up the channels of communication and feed cells. This is useful groundbreaking information. While this is complicated, the take home message is that an incredible process is in the making—a new millennium medicine.

GROWTH FACTORS — CELLULAR MESSENGERS

This developing area of medicine is hot. There is a lot here to learn, but getting the information under our belt is not easy. Pay attention, and I will lead you. There are four major growth factors: transforming growth factor (TGF-beta), insulin growth factor (IgF), Epidermal Growth Factor (EGF) and Platelet Derived Growth Factor (PDGF) We are most interested in TGF-beta for reasons that will soon become apparent.

Growth factors are a very special subset of circulating messengers collectively called cytokines, which make up the legion of craftsmen that are constantly involved in cell start-ups and cell destruction.

Transforming growth factor-beta (TGF-beta) is likely the most important: It is a master cytokine – one that controls hosts of other cytokines. An awareness of this research is stimulating considerable interest because of the immense potential it may have for the treatment of chronic degenerative diseases, especially those involving fibrosis and sclerosis. When tissues are scarring and hardening, it would be of tremendous importance if agents were available to put the brakes on the process. Agents that modify TGF-beta are captivating a craving audience.

We know that aging itself—not only disease—is characterized by these processes, so those interested in preserving youth are looking very carefully at growth factors, TGF-beta being the one that is at the center of discussion.

Research on TGF-beta was reviewed in the May 2, 2000 *New England Journal of Medicine*. Here is a synopsis of the findings:

- TGF-beta is a small biochemical protein that stimulates cell division and regeneration. It is an important member of a small class of compounds called growth factors.
- They are essential, particularly when you are forming in the womb, or sprouting up as a young lad or lady. You need just the right amount. Too much and you are a giant. Too little and you are a dwarf. This is the situation for the early part of your life.
- In later adulthood, something else begins to happen. We begin to age. Fibrosis, sclerosis, and hypercoagulability begin to occur. Adhesion molecules begin to appear in the circulation. They are regulated by growth hormones, particularly TGF-beta.
- For TGF-beta, the task is to assess the needs of the immune system for controlling inflammation and then to release specific cellular mediators, known as cytokines, in just the right amount to control inflammation and assure rapid and complete healing.

The recognition of growth factors and how they work is less than a decade old. It was in 1990 that Dr. A. B. Roberts and Dr. M. B. Sporn initially reviewed seminal work in a chapter called "The Transforming Growth Factors," appearing in the text were Peptide Growth Factors and Their Receptors.[1] In 1996, Drs. Roberts and Sporn updated the advancing knowledge, especially as these substances related to wound healing.[2] In 1999, a chapter was devoted to TGF-beta in the third edition of Gallin & Snyderman's textbook, *Inflammation*.[3] Then, in April 2000, Drs. C. E. Blobe, S. E. Schiemann, and F. M. Lodism published the review in what many consider the most prestigious medical journal in the world—*The New England Journal of Medicine*[4]. In this article, years of accumulated research from the Whitehead Institute for Biomedical Research in Cambridge, Massachusetts, Massachusetts Institute of Technology in Boston, Dana Farber Cancer Institute of New England, Department of Medicine from Massachusetts General Hospital and Harvard Medical School was presented.

So what does all this mean to us? It should excite us and stimulate us to learn more, because, perhaps this is the fertile path toward achieving longer and more youthful life. This is likely a very important path for the prevention or treatment of cancer, heart disease, kidney failure, and aging brain disorders.

In Europe, there is an increasing use of systemic oral enzyme therapy for many conditions, because one of the very important ways that this type of therapy works is by modulating cytokines, especially TGF-beta. What is clinically seen, and appreciated by the enthusiasts who regularly take enzymes, is that they heal quicker, have more energy, and do not seem to have early problems with heart disease, kidney disease, or cancer. When I was in Germany last spring, on the wall of a pharmacy at Maria Square in Munich there was a poster that said: Enzymes: Fitness for the Immune System. Absolutely true? Perhaps not. Kernel of valuable truth? I think so. Worth pursuing? Definitely!

We know more about TGF-beta because of the clinical investigations surrounding oral proteolytic enzymes and the various products that normalize their production: Wobenzym® N, Phlogenzym®, Wobe- Mugos®.

CLINICAL VIGNETTE #6

Mary Jo, a 44-year-old Caucasian female, has scleroderma, a disease that causes advancing fibrosis and sclerosis of nerves, arteries and mucus membranes. She has had persistent pain in the chest wall and joints. In spite of chemotherapy, her disease has been progressive.

Mary Jo was not doing well at all. She was looking for help. I placed her on a diet, stress reduction, and a supplement program. She was asked to eat fresh fruits and vegetables for breakfast, with a moderate amount of protein. She was to shift some of her carbohydrate load to the evening where the body was better able to handle it. She was asked to take vitamin E (400 IU a day), horse chestnut (400 milligrams in two divided doses daily) and Wobenzym® N (5 tablets twice a day). Her pain improved. She is now hopeful that her life—both quality and quantity—is going to be improved. Before the new therapy program, she thought that she was out of options. Her hope was slim and she felt that she just had to wait as her disease took her life. Now, perhaps, there is a future.

Scleroderma is a fibrosing disease, where we know that TGF-beta is increased. We do not understand the etiology and the pathogenesis of this disease very well. To date, no genetic linkage has been identified. But we do know that sclerosis is involved and agents that modify TGF-beta are potential agents that may help us prevent, arrest or reverse this disease.

CLINICAL VIGNETTE #7

Jannette is a 51-year-old Caucasian female with rheumatoid arthritis. She was on methotrexate, but it just drained her. She felt that it helped her arthritis, but she just didn't like all the side effects and the way that she felt when she was on this strong anti-cancer drug. She had stopped it on her own several months prior to visiting my office. She was placed on antioxidants, and told to increase her fluids, vitamins and enzymes. She was asked to go easy on the carbohydrates, especially the white starches. She began to take glucosamine sulfate (GS-500 at 1,500 mg a day) and the Wobenzym® N systemic oral enzyme combination before meals. What she noticed was that her joints became less swollen and her energy came up. Her labs were followed and both her C-reactive protein and her sedimentation rates became normal.

Rheumatoid arthritis causes severe, and often disabling arthritis. There is considerable fibrosis associated with this disease as scar tissue called pannus is laid into the joint spaces. There are also high levels of inflammatory proteins, most notably C-reactive protein. As we understand further the triggers and accelerated pathways of inflammation, prevention and reversal of this disease becomes more achievable.

Understanding cellular messaging is going to be very important. Cells must recognize what is self and what is not. The surveillance system must arrest—on the spot—early wildfires so that they do not scar the landscape. As millennium medicine advances, more answers are within our grasp.

THE METAPHOR

The tower of Babel is a familiar metaphor to anyone with even a cursory knowledge of early Biblical stories. When a group of men and women got together and tried to build a tower high into the clouds in an attempt to build a worldly access into heaven, it was seen as man's hubris or arrogance. God gave them all different languages so that they could not understand one other. The result was chaos. We must be humble—humble enough to learn to listen. Unless we listen to and learn the language of our cells, they will be babbling at one another, and subsequently not communicating successfully with each other and working together. Mounting a successful healing response will simply not occur unless this is accomplished.

BITTER ROOTS

THE PRINCIPLE

Our beliefs create a unique biology within us, which creates behavior. This relationship is cause and effect. It is equally true that changes in behavior cause changes in biology, which directly cause us to change our beliefs.

THE LAW

Optimize Healthy Beliefs & Behaviors. Expect Speedy Healing.

ENHANCEMENT

The concept presented here is simple enough: Your thoughts influence your health. Equally true is that your behavior—what you eat, how much you exercise, your sexual practices—influence health. Both of the following statements are equally true!

What you think and believe causes changes in your physiology.

Changes in your physiology cause changes in what you believe and think.

THE EMPHASIS

To reclaim salubrity, you must develop healthy thoughts. You must come to believe and understand what is normal and healthy. Your thoughts, your attitudes, and the very smile on your face can be trained to stay there.

Understand also that you can choose to eat a balanced diet, commit to a regular exercise program, adopt a regular sleeping pattern, and live an active, but balanced social life. Speedy health improvement will be the result, especially when accompanied by lightheartedness and a sense of humor.

DISCUSSION

When a problem occurs, traditional psychology teaches that understanding the problem will lead to a resolution of the problem. This is well and good, but it is only looking at one side of the playing field. This type of therapy—known as cognitive behavioral therapy—advocates that delving into reason will produce a healing response. If and when the reason is discovered and understood, healthy behavior will soon follow.

The father of cognitive behavior therapy was Sigmund Freud. The pervasive influence of Dr. Freud on the current practice of psychology and psychiatry cannot be overemphasized. This approach has defined the field of mental illness to merely "disturbances of interpretation" that lead to anxiety, neurosis, depression, agoraphobia, insomnia and the entire gamut of nonphysiological somatic complaints. While I believe Freud embodied genius, it is time to reframe, and move beyond, his perspective.

The flip side of this approach is known as behavioral cognitive therapy. The field of addiction medicine has championed this approach because when a person has very abnormal behavior, such as compulsive alcohol abuse, first and foremost this behavior needs to be stopped immediately. When the behavior is eliminated, the physiology gradually begins to return to normal. When a person enters an alcoholic rehabilitation program—usually a twelve-step program—a new and healthy identity emerges. It is as if the cocoon has been broken open.

The military has also advocated this approach. If you are lost, overweight, out-of-shape, broke and not knowing what you want to do in life, then come and join the army; be the best that you can be. This process, known as induction, is first and foremost behavioral. A person's outward appearance is changed with a haircut and a shave. New and conforming clothes are issued. A healthy diet is presented without options, and a rigorous schedule is laid out—there is no room for debate about where your time is going to be spent. What happens is that the new behavior changes the physiology and the beliefs of the inductee. After boot camp, a new identity emerges—a soldier is born.

MORE EXAMPLES: HOW BELIEFS & BEHAVIOR ARE INTERRELATED

Negative:

The National Health and Nutrition Examination Survey (NHANES-I) evaluated 5,007 women and 2,886 men who completed the database for the Center for Disease Control in 1982-84 and were known at that time to be free of coronary heart disease (hardening of the arteries)[5]. In the year 2000, the NHANES-I team reassessed these individuals. They were looking to see how many of these nearly 8000 individuals met criteria for clinical depression during the interim. They found that the adjusted relative risk for heart disease, when one had developed depression, was 173 percent for women and 171 percent for men compared to non-depressed individuals – an almost two fold risk increase.

There is overwhelming data that women who are sad, bitter, and carry the weight of the world in their breast have an increased incidence of cancer with more aggressive tumors.

Bad marriages, characterized by frequent emotional battles, anger, and despair lead to hypertension and heart disease in men.

Positive:

Interventional cognitive therapy is shown to be very effective through the work of O. Carl Simonton in his book *Getting Well Again*. Here, he demonstrated that structured positive imagery improved cancer survival: Good thoughts heal.

Studies of love within a stable long-term relationship have shown that we can expect a longer life span and the best of health. When marital relationships go sour, so does the health, even when diet and lifestyle changes are considered and statistically factored out.

In a behavioral oriented treatment center, based on a twelve-step program, persons with addiction disorder can be successfully treated. Laughter, especially when accompanied by deliberate playful activity, leads to rapid healing, both physical and emotional.

CLINICAL VIGNETTE #8

Peggy is now 17 years old. She is doing fairly well, but the last several years of her life have been transforming. In the summer and early fall of 1999, Peggy spent three months in a treatment center for adolescents with eating disorders. The situation at home had gotten out of control. She was five feet seven inches and her weight had dropped down to 84 pounds. The sodium in her blood had gotten dangerously low and her liver was showing signs of failure.

Eight months earlier, to be exact, the evening of December 5, 1998, Peggy's parents had discovered her throwing up in the bathroom during her shower after dinner. This behavior was confronted and abruptly stopped. By this time, it was clear that Peggy had bulimia, an eating disorder characterized by bingeing and regular vomiting after meals. The bulimic behavior had become strongly entrenched in Peggy's thoughts and actions. If the vomiting was not going to be allowed, Peggy's mind reasoned that she was not going to eat. She didn't. Her weight progressively dropped over the next six months even though she was seeing a nutritionist who had her on an exchange program and was seeing two different psychologists, both of whom seemed only interested in Peggy's early childhood experiences, which were not all that eventful. In Peggy's early childhood, there were a few issues to cling to—a new school at age twelve, having to make new friends, the perception that her parents argued constantly, threatening divorce, and an incident at camp where her peers made fun of her. While all these incidences were traumatic, at least in Peggy's eyes, their causal relationship to her eating disorder was doubtful. The cognitive behavioral therapy just wasn't working. The sessions likely got Peggy a little more talkative. The usual exercise of finger pointing was done—to her parents, her teachers, and her sib-

lings—but there was no stand-up ovation or catharsis of guilt, to ensure the eating disorder was chased away. A major breakthrough was not happening; the treatment was going nowhere.

When Peggy entered The Center for Change in Orem, Utah, the anorexic behavior was stopped immediately. She had a nasal gastric tube placed and she was fed and monitored twenty-four hours a day. Intensive group therapy was started and there was a lot of love around the center; she could feel it. Yet, most of the program was based on behavioral changes. If you ate, you got privileges. Peggy did—eventually—eat, and as her weight came up, her beliefs began to change. The world began to not seem so bleak. When Peggy left the center three months later, she looked and felt great. Her weight was 117 pounds and her appetite seemed pretty good until she got home. Peggy experienced some backsliding as the home environment was encountered. There were arguments regarding independence. Her parents monitored her eating and weight. There were a whole lot of tears.

Counseling was continued and so was group therapy. Yet, there were still tears. While the eating disorder was being held at bay, there was associated depression. The behavioral changes did not yet have sufficient strength to rid these thoughts. It was agreed that Peggy be placed on citalopram (Celexa) for depression. At a low dose, 20 mg a day, the tears dried up, and a higher level of health gradually followed. Peggy still struggles, but she is doing well today.

Eating disorders—anorexia nervosa and bulimia—are carving out a domain in adolescents. We need to wake up and help them focus on healthy beliefs regarding their bodies, even when their measurements are nowhere near that of Barbie or the Gap model on the wall of their favorite clothing store. If we want them to be healthy, we must insist that adequate and appropriate time be set aside for meals, especially family meals where most of their early ideas and behaviors originate. We need to go into our schools and insist that all grades, especially the first and second graders, be given adequate time to eat their lunches. What is learned well, early on, will persist and shape our futures. Let us do the same for our children.

THE METAPHOR

An anonymous sage said: "Bitter roots bear sour fruit." Extend your imagination to consider the behavior of a living tree and its ability to bear edible fruit. This is dependent on the actions of the roots as they go out seeking the right nourishment. Sometimes, it is right there; the farmer is providing the essentials immediately at the base of the tree. In the usual, not so fortunate situation, the roots have to go out looking. They extend themselves to, and beyond, a hundred feet to meet the needs of the living tree. Various nutrients are encountered. Choices have to be made. Imagine for a moment that roots are intelligent, and perhaps they are. What the roots believe will affect their choice—a behavioral choice. That choice will determine whether or not there is healthy fruit—divinely edible, salubrious fruit. That choice, if unhealthy, may cause there to be bitter fruit or no fruit. But if we can direct the roots to the most nutritious soils, then we can see the tree of life in all its glory and abundance. Behavior produces belief in all kingdoms upon Earth.

Principle & Law Eight
TOXIC PLANET

THE PRINCIPLE
Environment Induces Gene Expression.

THE LAW
Live in a Healthy Environment and Healing Happens.

ENHANCEMENT
Environment induces genetic changes. In a truly safe environment, illness will not occur—the Garden of Eden truism—but few of us find ourselves in such a benevolent garden.

The physical, emotional, mental, and spiritual body will be protected in a safe environment. The emphasis on milieu for maintaining health and enhancing healing cannot be over-emphasized. It takes a healthy family and a loving village to raise healthy children.

THE EMPHASIS
The environment can be highly toxic. Oxidation, one form of toxicity, results from free radical formation. Oxidation leads to changes in membranes, aberrations in our genetic materials, damages our cellular energy factories (i.e., mitochondria), and opens the door to a wide variety of dis-

eases. Some experts have suggested that oxidative stress may be the common pathway for all degenerative diseases.

DISCUSSION

Each cell in the human sustains up to 10,000 "hits" a day from free radicals, yet, somehow is able to stay intact and healthy. Our cells maintain their health through a comprehensive oxidative-reductive system whereby certain nutrients and buffers in the human body can sustain and absorb the hit—at least when we are healthy. Not only are there physical hits from the outside environment but there are also internally generated hits. Our thoughts and our emotions generate cortisol, adrenaline, and other vasoconstrictors which can then shift our metabolism into higher glucose demand, higher acidity in the internal environment and hence, more free radical damage.

When poisons penetrate, our vulnerability to illness increases. Changes in physiology occur and aberrant cellular behavior begins. In fact, our genetic expression will change; changes in circulating levels of RNA transcriptase can even be seen.

We need to identify these external and internal detonators. If we can, we need to shield ourselves. Sunscreen protects the skin against ultraviolet radiation, and the herb milk thistle protects the liver against some chemical toxins.

The focus of scientific investigation has recently seen a mild shift toward studying mitochondrial DNA and its susceptibility to oxidative stress. It is now appreciated that our weakest link may be the cell membrane, which is so vitally important as a shield. If the cell membrane has been breached, the DNA is at risk of sustaining damage. When this happens, our energy factories, located in the mitochondria, are damaged and we become ill.

The work of Linus Pauling and his colleagues, most notably Jeff Bland, Ph.D., continues to advance knowledge in this area through the Institute of Functional Medicine. It is likely that oxidative stress is the major killer of our cell membranes and causally linked to DNA damage and chronic disease. As we understand this concept more fully, a major lock and key mechanism will be available to us to more effectively reclaim and preserve health.

THE METAPHOR

Generations of *Star Trek* fans have viewed the rings of toxic planets. Ours is becoming one and in a not so far away time, our planet may well become uninhabitable because of this toxicity. On the positive note, advances in antioxidant stress management are surging. Linus Pauling relied on vitamins C and E—but there is a new wave of very popular and powerful antioxidants: pycnogenol, grapeseed extract, selenium, beta-glucan, and proven herbomineral formulas such as GeriCare® (also known as Geriforte® worldwide).

The issue of oxidative stress has achieved widespread acceptance, even among very conservative physicians. As individuals seeking salubrity strengthen their antioxidant health management programs, the results will surely be gratifying.

Principle & Law Nine

WALLS OF JERICO

THE PRINCIPLE

Our physical body and energetic force fields must be fortified, or else they will crumble like the walls of Jericho.

THE LAW

Enhance the Defense to Augment the Healing Response.

ENHANCEMENT

An arsenal of builders must be present, trained, and ready to rebuild. There are a host of threats that continually tear away at the structure of our bodies. These insults are not just physical, but may be emotional and mental. We must continually build and repair the home defenses. A healthy home is a beautiful and essential fortress. Vitamins, minerals, herbs, antioxidants and enzymes are key defenders.

THE EMPHASIS

There is structure and there is function. Make sure the building blocks are available to your body so that the machinery of rebuilding is always bustling.

DISCUSSION

Arthritis is "fire in the joints." Such a sensation is surely one that we would like to avoid. If avoiding the onset of arthritis is potentially one of the "I wish I had known" lessons learned too late, there is good news. If we step in early with measures that stop the wear and tear of our joints, we can decrease or eliminate further damage or pain from arthritis.

Arthritis is not the result of aging; it is the result of degeneration of the cartilage in your joints. Older individuals get it more often than younger people, but this isn't always true. It is associated with, and not just caused by, the passing of time.

Arthritis may follow trauma, because sudden impacts can certainly harm cartilage. If proper care and healing is not allowed to occur, arthritis will develop. Runners may be prone to arthritis, but this is usually because of multiple traumas; running does not cause arthritis. Running is fine, but you have to wear good shoes and run only within the context of an exercise program that is balanced with flexibility and strengthening.

Being overweight and out of shape certainly can set the stage for arthritis, but the issue is not so much the weight, as the health of the supporting tissue. Weight is toxic to your system—especially if you cannot support it. This means that if you have strong muscles, tendons, and ligaments, it is likely you will have healthy joints.

Having good circulation is also essential. If you don't get your aerobics—daily uninterrupted, heart-targeted exercise—your tissues will ache. Your body needs rich, precious, free flowing, oxygenated blood, filled with life-giving nutrients, to stay healthy. Without this, toxic products will accumulate and tear down the fortress.

Dehydration is toxic; hydration is crucial to avoid arthritis. Are you consuming six to eight glasses of fresh water per day, or do you think that the six-pack of diet Coke or Coors is the same thing?

The bitter cold is not toxic to your joints and does not cause arthritis, although it will amplify the pain and stiffness. It is the rapid changes in barometric pressure that affect joints.

Mental stress does not cause arthritis. We can't blame our emotions for everything. If you are an individual who is always in the fight-or-flight mode, you are expending too much extra adrenalin. This is unsettling to your health. Adrenalin will cause blood vessels to spasm, make you jittery, and interrupt your sleep. Pain perception can increase. Mental stress may not cause arthritis but it can certainly make things worse.

It is likely that low levels of toxins in the environment such as lead, mercury and arsenic, as well as continuous exposure to pesticides and irradiation—and even biological pathogens—are either causative or aggravating factors.

We know that we have to be strong in order to stay healthy. Wear and tear is as real as the air we breathe. Toxins, allergens and various intruders are always working on our joints: They are breaking them down. Hence, it is necessary to always have on hand adequate rebuilding materials and to continually be sure that inflammation is not able to get a chronic grip.

The following recommendations are prudent for structural support:
Glucosamine sulfate (500 mg, three times daily)
Calcium citrate (400 to 800 mg daily)
Magnesium (300 to 400 mg daily)
Manganese (3 mg daily)
Boron (3 mg daily)
Methyl sulfonylmethane or MSM (1,000 mg, three times daily)
For functional support, especially as it relates to controlling chronic inflammation and keeping scarring to a minimum, consider the following:
Systemic oral enzymes (Wobenzym® N, five tablets, three times daily)
Horse chestnut seed extract (30 mg, twice daily)

CLINICAL VIGNETTE #9
Michael is a 49-year- old baby boomer with baby boomer blessings he sees as problems—a nagging, overly strict wife, five kids (all daughters), and financial uncertainty. Getting the daily tasks done is hard enough, but keeping the muscle and fat where it is supposed to be is a never-ending task.

Michael has had two knee surgeries from basketball trauma about ten years ago. In fact, the initial trauma involved a compression fracture to the medial femoral condyle (i.e., he wrecked the cartilage and bone in the medial compartment of the right knee). He put on about 12 pounds after surgery and hasn't been able to get it off.

Previously, he relied on running to sort of fix his weight when it would start to go up. Now, depressed, stiff, and unable to run, there does not seem to be an easy answer.

Part of the answer came when Michael started taking glucosamine sulfate. There was less pain, less barometric pressure, and a better ability to move about. In fact, with time, the pain in the knee went away entirely on glucosamine sulfate therapy. But running? This was not even a consideration. There did not seem to be even a remote possibility that this would ever happen.

Michael then started taking systemic oral enzyme therapy on a regular basis (Wobenzym® N). This regimen was necessary to be sure that any microtrauma did not result in having to stop the exercise program. The results were extraordinary. Not only did Michael start running five miles on the treadmill (no elevation yet), but he also was running nine–and sometimes eight-minute miles three times a week. His weight has dropped by 10 pounds. The stiffness is minimal to none. The pain in the knee is gone. Appetite is good but not excessive. Energy is up.

Maintaining super nutrient status is important. Our diets are just not adequate. Over 55 percent of Americans are obese and 22 percent are considered morbidly obese (greater than 20 percent overweight). We are not eating our fresh fruits and vegetables. If we eat them at all on a daily basis, it is likely that preservatives have been sprayed on them or pesticides have been used to boost their yield. (Have you looked at the size of strawberries lately?) Worse, vegetables are often radiated—with cobalt—to extend their shelf life. We are moving farther and farther away from natural foods towards more variety and more convenience.

THE METAPHOR

The tumbling walls of Jericho: In the book of Joshua, the Lord instructed the horns to be blown around the city for seven days at which time the walls of the city would fall. They did.When did your body's walls begin to tumble? Did the horn blow on your 39th birthday? I hope not.

Principle & Law Ten

LOST LAMB FOUND

THE PRINCIPLE

Connectedness to God, according to your understanding, positively influences your health and aging. Having spiritual health will slow the rate of aging and dramatically lower incidence of many diseases.

THE LAW

Slow aging and accelerate healing by filling the well of your spiritual reservoir.

ENHANCEMENT

The issue behind Principle and Law Ten—spirituality and healing—is so basic, so fundamental, and so foundational, that its simplicity seems to escape us: Spiritual health is important. The concept must embrace connectedness to God, according to your understanding. To sidestep, and attempt to appease agnostics and atheists, does health and healing a disservice. It essentially negates the idea that there are positive influences in the energetic connectedness to higher energies outside of ourselves.

Your identity is composed of physical, mental, emotional, social and spiritual relationships. To live long, maintain your health, and attain your dreams depends on your security within your unique identity.

Centenarians will tell you time and again that love, family, friends, and a stable relationship with God are core essentials to seemingly ageless living. Optimal—*enviable health*—requires a connectedness to God (or as members of Alcoholics Anonymous would express: "to your Higher Power as you have come to understand Him or Her"). We must develop a reverence for this connectedness, and not be distracted by negative past experiences. The language of spiritual health, the language that heals, is called prayer.

The Language of Connectedness

Spirit: The Unseen Self is our core identification—what we know to be our real being. This is the unique part of the energetic you that can transcend and bridge beyond the physical. It is operationally distinct from vital force because it is not relationally defined by ability to do work—although it can, as in an awakening whereby shame and blame are shed by freely granting forgiveness and letting spiritual love be unleashed. The spirit is distinct from the social or relational aspects of health, in that the focus of spiritual health is on connectedness to God, and the transcendent or miraculous healing power that is available through this connection. The spirit is distinct from the "soul"—at least in this context—only because the term "soul" is too much enshrined in theology and best left to religious scholars, with the exception of medical philosophers.

God: The English word most commonly used for the creator of the universe, and source of all absolute power is "God." Members of Alcoholics Anonymous refer to God as "The Higher Power." Larry Dossey, M.D., in his classic work on the power of prayer, *Healing Words*, prefers to avoid the word "God" and uses instead "The Absolute." Choose alternatively, if you wish. After all, free choice exists (Principle #1).

Prayer: The language of the communication with God. The word comes from the Latin "precari," meaning to entreat earnestly. Prayer may also involve confessing, or simply talking in one's own personal way. Prayer is not the same thing as meditation. In meditation, attention is directed inward, toward quieting the spirit. Communicating with God during meditation would be an expansion of the generally accepted definition. It is important to note that meditation, especially transcendental medication, will elicit, as will prayer, powerful calming and healing responses.

Miracle: An unusual happening, often a healing, not explained by traditional medicine, and which cannot be explained even by one of the many disciplines of alternative or complementary medicine. A miracle happens when God intervenes to provide it. God does miracles. He probably does a lot of them. Whether God has one for you is not something that another person can determine. It is up to you to ask and to be open and aware of its occurrence when it happens. It may not happen in the way that you expect. If or when the miracle happens, be sure to be thankful.

THE EMPHASIS

Talk to God. Ask God what you need to do every moment. That is what is meant by "pray with unceasing fervor." Request prayer from others. Be connected to your friends, family, and to God. Prayer opens up channels of non-localizing healing energy. It births the transcendent miraculous power available from God.

DISCUSSION

We are not sure why you, your friends, or a relative develops cancer, accelerated arthritis, heart disease, chronic obstructive lung disease, or a severe depression that leads to despair or even suicide. We are not sure why you feel older or your skin looks older than your classmates or your spouse, when perhaps you are, in fact, younger. However we do know more than we did ten to twenty years ago. Having a healthy spiritual vitality is a good thing—a transcendent quality that people notice. It is the smile on the face, and the inner peace that reveals that the spirit is vibrant. When this occurs, positive health is evident.

Having a locked down, constricted spirit is the opposite of a healthy vibrant spirit. When a lock down is occurring, healing can be very difficult.

Life deals out many challenges—or "wounds," as Caroline Myss, PH.D., calls them. When the wound is allowed to sustain or grow, a negative shell blocks spiritual pathways of healing. The person with a blocked spirit may even develop a unique language called "woundology," and communicate socially through this language. When wounded, individuals are entrenched with members of their support group, and their wounds are often validated, sometimes so much so that the healing response is blunted. Well-intentioned comfort has a time element, which must be recognized. Moving out and beyond the wounds takes courage. Change is fearful. In fact, psychological research shows that one fears death less than one fears change.

The key to healing individuals with a blocked spirit is to recognize what is happening and then gently begin turning their ship—perhaps a little at first, just enough to catch a bit of the wind that heals. A healing journey begins.

CLINICAL VIGNETTE #10

Peter was 42 years old. He was running his own professional business, and feeling pretty good about it. He diligently searched for an office manager who could effectively take over some of the business tasks. This way, Peter reasoned, he could give his full attention to seeing patients, and not be hampered by looking at insurance reimbursements and accounts receivables. For a while, things seemed great. The money came in and the books balanced. Connie, the office manager, seemed to like her job and seemed to be efficient.

Then, some things started to change. Connie seemed a little distant. She eventually admitted she was pregnant, not happy about it and feeling nauseated most of the time. Even though inefficiencies became noticeable, Peter backed off, and let well enough alone. After all, the pregnancy was not going well, and confrontation just did not seem the right thing to do.

During the time Connie took off to deliver a healthy baby boy, an office assistant and Peter's wife came in to do the books. It didn't take long to realize that Connie had been embezzling. She had stolen $3,000, but had also messed up the books by another $10,000. The situation was so bad that it was impossible to figure out what patients actually owed. It was embarrassing and, to add salt to the wound, Peter's wife, in her opinion, was being forced to come in to straighten things out.

The burden of anger was heavy. Peter fumed every time he thought about Connie. Being let down like this was depressing, and a spiritual weight of unforgiveness was upon him like a non-healing scab.

Peter knew that forgiving was a form of spiritual unburdening. But forgiving in the mind is very different than forgiving in person. About a year after the embezzlement, Peter got on the elevator in the basement of an industrial building and pushed the sixth floor button on his way to a workmen's compensation hearing. The door of the elevator opened on the first floor and Connie stepped in by herself. She pushed the second floor button. In an instant—less than five seconds, Peter said, "Connie, I forgive you for what you did."

Connie looked at Peter, a little baffled.

"Thank you," she replied, and got out on the second floor.

Peter felt a little dazed, and amazed at what he had just done. The result was awesome. It was instantaneous. The burden lifted. Spiritual healing occurred and the wound disappeared. To date, Peter never thinks about this anymore. There is absolutely no anger or bad feeling. It was like an eraser had removed the sore.

So what do we know about spiritual healing?

○ Too much attachment to the world takes away degrees of freedom. Sharing is good for our health. Being spiritually connected brings a harmony of mind and body. Individuals with an active prayer life are known to have decreased incidences of various medical problems including hypertension, heart disease and cancer.

○ Forgiveness opens up energy blockages. When one forgives, a spiritual event occurs, especially when it is face to face, and the listener acknowledges the forgiveness. A burden lifts and the spirits soar.

○ Positive imagery especially within the language of prayer is very powerful, especially when done in the context of the family and group prayer.

- We don't want to be lost. We need to have a purpose. When we have one, we can assume an amazing healing potential.
- Chronic pain syndrome is closely linked to the loss of identity, and the development of a reclusive life. When identity restructuring is done, and the self is rebuilt, the pain syndrome decreases.

What do we know about prayer and healing?

In Larry Dossey's *Healing Words*, the early research on prayer was reviewed up to at least 1993 when the book was published. In his preface, he notes that, "I found an enormous body of evidence. There were over one hundred experiments exhibiting the criteria of 'good science.' Many of these were conducted under stringent laboratory conditions. Over half of these studies showed that prayer brings about significant changes not only in people, but in a variety of living beings. These studies varied in design and scope, but were able to show that prayer positively influences multiple aspects of physiology."

- Blood pressure was lowered.
- Wounds healed more quickly.
- Heart attacks were less frequent and less severe.
- Enzymatic reactions were stimulated.
- Fungi growth rates were reduced.
- Bacteria grew more slowly.
- Cancer cells grew more slowly.
- Cardiac pacemaker cells were less irritable.
- Seeds grew more rapidly.
- Algae, moth larvae, mice and chicks growth rates were affected.

What must we do to begin spiritual healing?

- Be open to examining your spiritual self.
- Be willing to make some changes.
- Understand the powerful burdens and blockages you may have chosen to carry.

- Understand that there are people out there that can help you begin a healthy spiritual walk.
- Understand that nothing worthwhile is easy at first. It is like the athlete in training. Most will tell you that the most difficult part of their program is getting their shoes on and getting out the door.

THE METAPHOR

The lost sheep is seen as wandering and disconnected. The little one is away from the flock and the shepherd that protects it. When the sheep wanders, there are no defenses. There is extreme vulnerability.

Are we like the lost sheep? Do we have a macho façade? Do we have friends that support us, and lift us up? Do we seek to know God? How is our spiritual health? It is a rare few that could survive life as a hermit—without God.

Assessing Your Healing Response
STARTING YOUR PROGRAM

EACH OF THE TEN PRINCIPLES AND LAWS address health issues in a practical way that may or may not be of personal importance to you. If you are absolutely healthy, send this book on to a friend who needs it. If not, do a personal assessment, and examine whether your healing response is in an optimal state of preparedness.

20 ASSESSMENT TOOLS
1 **Get a physical exam.** Have your weight and height checked against standard life insurance tables. In fact, for fun, try applying for a million dollars worth of life insurance. You'll learn a lot. You will have to fill out a lot of questionnaires. Measurements will be obtained and reviewed by the risk management team of the insurance company who will clearly let you know whether you "measure up."

2 **Request a blood and urine analysis**. Specifically see that a complete blood count, a comprehensive metabolic profile, a urine exam, a thyroid panel and an ultra-sensitive thyroid stimulating hormone is done. The cost is less than a hundred dollars. These tests used to be routine in any physical examination—emphasis *"used to be."*

3 **Get a 24 hour urine analysis for toxic metals—lead, arsenic, and mercury**. Another, less reliable way to assure that you are not heavy metal toxic is to

have a hair analysis done. Take a clump of fairly new hair from the nape of your neck—enough to fill a teaspoon—and send it to the lab where toxic metal amounts will be assessed. Iron, another toxic metal, can also build up in your system. Iron overload, called hemachromatosis, is not uncommon, and it is a good idea to be tested for this illness which literally can rust your system. The test, a serum ferritin, is readily available. Have it done.

4 **Get dunked—the practice of being weighed underwater.** This is to assess percent body fat. Getting dunked has become quite popular at health clubs and the usual standards for men are betweem 12 to 17 percent body fat and for women, 15 to 23 percent is acceptable. One way to tell if you are in the ballpark is to get into the deep end of your pool, and see if you float with your lungs full of air. If you do not, and in fact sink with lungs full of air, you are probably less than 15 percent body fat. If you have to blow out your lung air and then sink, you are probably between 15 to 20 percent body fat—not bad. If you blow out all your air and you still float, your body fat is too high. Get active! Do something about it!

5 **Detox!** This refers to therapeutic programs whereby toxic waste is elimi-nated from your system. The most common way is to do it through the gastrointestinal tract, by going on a juice fast, such as carrot juice. There are multiple other programs whereby a simplified diet is combined with various detoxification products. These generally contain enzymes, antiox-idants, vitamins, high fiber, and often oral or intravenous chelators. Detoxification can be aided with purgatives and colonics, but often these methods can be too harsh. There are also programs that purge the gall bladder, and empty the liver of various toxins. The liver excretes by three pathways: mono-oxidation, conjugation, and the P450 enzyme system. All of these pathways can be accelerated or slowed down if desired. In any detoxification program, caution is advised. Get an understanding of what problems you have and be sure to find a knowledgeable practitioner if you are going to embark on a rigorous program. Choose a physician that is trained in functional medicine (fxmed.com), or an experienced naturo-pathic or holistic physician.

6 **Check your stress profile.** There are multiple events in our lives that will stress us out considerably, and we need to be aware of these. Look in the Glossary under Holmes-Rahe Social Readjustment Rating Scale. If you score over 300, you have an 80 percent chance of becoming seriously ill in the next year.

7 **Get a traditional oriental medicine assessment.** This should be fun because most traditional practitioners will check the strength, rhythm, and position of your twelve pulses (you probably didn't know you had that many). They will also check your tongue and check for tender points and then correlate them with acupuncture points. They may do an akabani meridian balance assessment. You will also find that the type of history taken will be very different. It will include an assessment of the effect of adverse influences such as wind, dry heat, and dampness. The treatment plan will likely include foods, herbs and an acupuncture program.

8 **Get checked by a homeopathic physician.** Call this another adventure, in that homeopathic physicians think a little differently than traditional physicians. They are very energy minded, and also pay attention to very minute details as they attempt to find a remedy for you

9 **Have your environment checked.** Did you know that carbon monoxide monitors are cheap and should be placed in any home where gas is used for cooking or heat? Air quality tests are available for your home. To improve the environmental health of your bedroom, it is a good idea to get a new mattress and new pillows every few years. Perhaps, when you get new tires on your car, change your pillows and mattresses. If you cannot afford these changes, at least flip your mattresses. Dust mites are very real and they accumulate in your pillows and in the superficial layers of your mattress. They are very allergenic, especially their excrement, which builds up and doesn't clean out well.

10 **Do basal body testing.** The thyroid gland regulates your general metabolism. It is fueling virtually every cell of your body through the mitochondrial phosphate mechanisms. Deficiencies of thyroid hormone are often very subtle and go unnoticed. When left unchecked, they progress and impact negatively on your health. Basal Body Temperature is the most sen-

sitive functional test of thyroid function. Body temperature reflects the underlying metabolic rate. To measure it, all you need is a thermometer. Your basal body temperature should be between 97.6 and 98.2 degrees Fahrenheit. When it is low, you are likely hypothyroid which causes fatigue, low energy and a host of symptoms you would rather not have. When it is high, you may be hyperthyroid, which causes hyperirritability, inability to gain weight, insomnia, menstrual problems, and weakness. Be sure to avoid some foods that can prevent the utilization of iodine and can cause hypothyroidism. These foods are termed goitrogens and include turnips, cabbage, mustard, cassava root, soybean, peanuts, pine nuts, and millet. Cooking usually inactivates goitrogens. Get plenty of exercise in that this is critical in stimulating thyroid gland secretions and increasing tissue sensitivity to thyroid hormone. Many health benefits from exercise may in fact result from improved thyroid function. This is especially important for overweight hypothyroid individuals.

11 **Check your heart and circulatory health.** There are various static and functional tests available that do not require an angiogram. For starters, take a walk. Choose a cool day, on a level surface for starters. See how far you can go and how long it takes. Better yet, get an exercise treadmill test done through your physician. If you really want to go all out, book a flight to Dallas and get tested at Ken Cooper's Aerobics Center. There, you can measure your "aerobic capacity." Getting your lipids tested is important. But rather than just getting your cholesterol measured, it is important to get the whole lipid profile, including an apolipoprotein A test, which gives an indication of hereditary risk of having a heart attack. Another very useful test is called The Heart Test, which is also referred to as the calcium heart test. This test uses high-speed sonography to look for calcium deposits in the heart's blood vessels. Certainly a diagnostic treadmill is easy enough: This can be followed by a thallium treadmill, or what is called multigated gallium treadmill (MUGA) test. Also, the next time you go in for a cholesterol check-up, ask your doctor to have a C-reactive protein (CRP) test performed. Measuring serum CRP levels can provide addi-

tional information on if your risk is high for a heart attack or stroke due to subacute inflammation. The test is now considered routine and relatively inexpensive (about fifty dollars).

12 **Have an oxidative stress test.** Urine and blood tests are available that can assess oxidative stress in your system. You may need more antioxidants.

13 **Check your white blood cells both quantitatively and qualitatively.** There are various types of white blood cells: granulocytes, lymphocytes, eosinophils, monocytes, and basophils. These numbers will be given on a complete blood count with differential. What is most interesting is to begin checking out the subsets and how various cells in the subsets respond to mitogen stimulation. Research regarding Acquired Immunodeficiency Syndrome (AIDS) has really bolstered our ability to assess the warehouses of the immune system and their functional readiness.

14 **Have quantitative and functional allergy testing.** This is another series of blood tests, looking at immunoglobulins, especially IgE and IgA subsets that are part of acute allergy symptoms. Hypersensitivity skin testing, known as "scratch testing," is also useful in some cases, especially in those individuals with chronic nasal congestion. If you are suffering from these types of problems, participating in a doctor supervised desensitization program can be very beneficial. Chronic food allergies are frequently mediated by IgG antibodies. If you have IgG antibodies to food, you can re-establish tolerance to these foods, if you are careful to avoid them for about three months and then slowly reintroduce them.

15 **Test for yeast overgrowth.** There are various questionnaires which may be helpful to assess risk. There are laboratory analyses that are also helpful: specific candida antibody and candida immune complex testing.

16 **Assay your hormones.** There is considerable literature that correlates dehydroepiandrosterone (DHEA) levels with aging. When your DHEA level is too low, you will age more quickly. Be sure to have your DHEA-sulfate level measured. Also important is to have both men *and* women measure their body's production of testosterone. The role of testosterone in women is underestimated; their bodies require it as well. Equally impor-

tant is to measure estrogen levels, which can be done with a twenty-four hour urine test. Another option, recently more fashionable, is to have salivary estrogen levels measured—known as "spit testing." Check your calcium levels, and correlate these with parathyroid hormone levels to assess whether you are at risk for osteoporosis. Check your prolactin levels which if elevated mean that pituitary function is going down. Have a vitamin D test done. This will be helpful if you are at risk for skin cancer in that this vitamin has considerable protective effects against cancer in general, and this cancer in particular.

17 **Assay your body's vitamin and mineral levels.** There are various labs that will check for every vitamin. The most important are folic acid and vitamin B_{12}. A deficiency of folic acid has been associated with increased cancer risk in adults, and neural tube defects in offspring. Low B_{12} levels are known to be the cause of pernicious anemia and various forms of dementia, most notably, the Wernicke Korsakoff Syndrome, commonly seen in alcoholics.

18 **Blow into the lung machine.** Basic lung function testing is called spirometry and measures the vital capacity of your lungs—along with their volumes and elasticity (which is your ability to blow out most of your air within one second). Other fairly simple tests measure lung volumes and lung residuals. These will help assess your risk of early emphysema or asthma.

19 **Get a preventive cancer examination.** In women, the most important exams are those of the breast and colon. For men, it is important to have colon, prostate, and lung exams. Postmenopausal women should have annual or biannual mammograms along with regular monthly breast self-examinations. For colon cancer, check the stool for blood, and get a sigmoidoscopy or colonoscopy (a sigmoidoscopy checks only the left colon, whereas the colonoscopy checks the whole colon). For anyone with a family history of abdominal or pelvic cancers, an abdominal sonogram should be considered to look for masses in the liver, kidney, or ovaries. Scoping the uterus, or getting a lavage for cytology, is sometimes recommended. Scoping the bladder is important if there is any blood in the urine (do not

always assume that a little blood is a little bit of an infection). The prostate specific antigen (PSA) test is useful for prostate cancer and prostatic ultrasound has found some favor. The carcinoembryonic antigen (CEA) test is useful for ovarian and some types of liver cancer. A serum protein electrophoresis can help detect multiple myeloma.

20 Assess the anatomy and readiness of your spirit. This is a very individual assessment in that you must look within to understand your unseen self, and then look without to see how you relate to your universe and the God that created you. If you are lost and connected only to the material bridge of your estate, you must gather the courage to find another individual to help you begin your spiritual path.

10 ORGANIZERS & 10 PEARL SUPPLEMENTS

An anonymous well-wisher once told me that the hardest part of any exercise program is getting on your shoes—followed by getting out the door. In my experience with both my patients and myself, I have found this to be absolutely true. So here is what I want you to do. Copy or cut this page from your book and put it on the refrigerator door and date when each of these important milestones is reached.

10 Organizers

1	Get a daily calendar	Date Achieved: _____
2	Organize home and office	Date Achieved: _____
3	Buy basic quality supplements	Date Achieved: _____
4	Select an accountability friend	Date Achieved: _____
5	Join health club	Date Achieved: _____
6	Obtain perfect training shoes	Date Achieved: _____
7	Make appointment with holistic doctor	Date Achieved: _____
8	Find right web sites	Date Achieved: _____
9	Locate the neigborhood health food store	Date Achieved: _____
10	Finish *The Healing Response*	Date Achieved: _____

10 Reliable Supplements to Strongly Consider

1 **Glucosamine sulfate.** Together with Drs. Megan Shields and Gary Wikholm, I co-authored *Arthritis: The Doctor's Cure* (Keats 1998), which focused heavily on a formula called **GS-500** from Enzymatic Therapy or **Glucosamine Sulfate** from PhytoPharmica. We have not changed our minds. For joint health with pure glucosamine sulfate, this is the premiere brand. Use it.

2 **Systemic oral enzymes.** Together with medical journalist David W. Steinman, I authored *The Aspirin Alternative* (Freedom Press 1999). This book reported on the European **Wobenzym®N** systemic oral enzyme formula available in America through Naturally Vitamins. Combine **Wobenzym®N** with glucosamine sulfate for a powerful overall joint health support program. Take five **Wobenzym® N** tablets twice daily on an empty stomach.

3 **Garlic.** For super vitality, take one tablet of **Garlinase-4000** by Enzymatic Therapy every day. Garlic is excreted through the skin, naturally cleansing it and helps reduce bothersome yeast in the gastrointestinal tract.

4 **Vitamin C.** Take at least one gram of vitamin C, twice daily. Vitamin C is one of the most important dietary supplements for cancer and heart disease prevention, as well as healthy teeth and gums. If stomach upset is a problem with large doses, a form of neutralized vitamin C should be used to avoid such problems. Look for vitamin C products bound to calcium or products containing Ester-C.

5 **MSM.** For joint pain, methylsulfonyl methane has also been very helpful. Make sure your brand is **Opti-MSM** from Cardinal Nutrition for added purity. Take one to five grams daily.

6 **Barlean's Lignan Rich Flax Oil**. For receiving adequate supplies of omega-3 fatty acids, there is no brand better than Barlean's. Use their capsules or take a tablespoon daily. Flax can be used for baking and in salad dressings.

7 **Magnesium.** Supplemental magnesium is essential to many dimensions of your well being. A healthy heart, muscles, nerves, and bowels all depend on it. If you are on pain medications, especially opioids, which

tend to constipate, magnesium supplements will usually normalize the bowels. I have found that the most reliable product in my hands has always been **Slow-Mag** (Slow Release Magnesium Chloride) by Roberts Labs in Eatonville, New Jersey. Another worthy product is **Wake-Up Insurance** from Age Smart. There are various salts of magnesium that may have added benefit. For fibromyalgia, mag-malic may be preferred. For memory problems, mag-taurine.

8 **IP$_6$ with Inositol.** Use the Enzymatic Therapy or PhytoPharmica brand of this important anti-cancer pill.

9 **Coenzyme Q$_{10}$.** Take 90 mg daily for overall cardiovascular and periodontal health, as well as cancer prevention. This is the key metabolic cofactor for the body's energy production.

10 **Probiotics.** These supply beneficial strains of bacteria to enhance gastrointestinal health. Select from among the following companies and you will be on solid ground because of the research that backs up their products: Enzymatic Therapy, Natural Factors, Wakunaga of America (i.e., Kyo-Dophilus), Nutrition Now, and Jarrow. **Prebiotics** supply essential nutrients to build up the beneficial flora. Search out a reliable inulin product with added fructo-oligosaccharides. **InuFlora**™ is a proprietary source of inulin derived from Jerusalem artichoke fiber. For further information on this, read *The Healing Power of Jerusalem Artichoke Fiber* which I authored, and was published by Freedom Press (freedompressonline.com).

FROM DR. LOES—WITH LOVE

LET IT BE EMPHASIZED THAT THE TEN PRINCIPLES and laws of healing are offered as a personal guide to you for taking either small starting steps or taking a quantum leap. Your health depends on it.

Whatever happens to us, the healing response of the energetic body—*mind, emotion and spirit*—will respond. The healing response, when enhanced, will engage. All it can muster will be produced. The healing response is not like the "fight or flight" reaction, because when it comes to healing, there is no flight. We engage in the battle for our life. There is no escaping, except into death, which we all hope is a long way away in the distant future.

We must learn to respect and trust our healing response. It is uniquely ours. Perhaps, today, you may not be sure how strong yours is, though you likely have some idea of its strength. If your healing response is weaker than optimal, it's time to direct your efforts toward enhancing it.

Our task today is to help you be prepared. You need to listen and learn. Your body speaks to you—your gut reaction is real. What is learned must be followed by action. This means that unhealthy thoughts and behaviors must be changed.

The healing response is not a myth; it is a vital reality. We have explained to you this health-achieving response in energetic terms because we are not just a clump of immobile clay, but moving, living beings. We are not just bricks and mortar that need a patch here or a paste there, as many physicians would like to think of us. Being alive is having energy in motion. Our loved ones are the *light and energy*, of our lives. We live. We love. We interact. Let us live together in salubrity, achieving and maintaining that "state of enviable health." We all want that. Be bold. Reclaim enviable health.

SPECIAL SECTIONS

Pain & Depression

THE HEALING RESPONSE

Pain is an individually unpleasant sensory, emotional and perceptual experience caused by actual tissue damage or described in terms of such damage.

PAIN IS UNPLEASANT. Few would disagree with this statement, except perhaps those decathlon athletes who somehow find pain exhilarating. Pain can consume you – dragging down all aspects of the energetic you. We must learn to understand it better. Pain has different energetic dimensions, and if you take a moment to checklist your symptoms from the chart below, this will be an important step.

SYMPTOMS OF PAIN:
UNHEALTHY IN BODY, EMOTIONS, MIND & SPIRIT:

	Physical		*Emotional*		*Mental*		*Spiritual*
I have	Pain; it hurts!	*I feel*	Sad	*I can't*	Think	*I'm*	Detached
I can't	Walk, Eat		Angry		Listen		Friendless
	Have Sex		Bitter		Watch		Alone
	Work		Nervous		Count		Bored
	Urinate		Agitated		Focus		Listless
	Move Bowels		Drained		Hear		Guilty
	Lie Still		Unloved		Sleep		Unsaved

As an internist who specializes in the evaluation of patients with pain and addiction problems, I have an immense challenge. I see one individual at a time and listen to their pain. I inquire when and how it began. I gently search out possible explanations on the elusive "Why do I have Pain?" question. I listen and permit the patient to talk without interruption. Research has shown that the average physician listens to a patient for only 17 seconds before they interrupt and start jumping to conclusions. Physicians need to become listeners. Patients are crying to be heard.

The Physical

It is important to determine, as best as possible, which physical structure in the body is generating the pain and which neurological pathway(s) are involved. For muscle and bone pain, there are basically three ways in which they generate pain – by thermal, chemical, or mechanical irritants. This means that excessive heat, irritating chemicals and abnormal mechanical forces – stretching, crushing, breaking – cause the pain and the accompanying inflammation. In medical jargon, muscle/bone pain is called nociceptive because these "noise receptors" are firing. They may be firing on the exterior of the body, as in muscles or bones, or "inside" as in the viscera (the guts).

Traditionally, non-steroidal anti-inflammatory agents (NSAIDs) are used to treat physical pain from muscle and bones. Many of the drugs are familiar to us—ibuprofen (Advil), naproxen (Aleve), and the more expensive, newer agents, known as COX-2 inhibitors: celecoxib (Celebrex) and rofecoxib (Vioxx). As a group, these agents are widely prescribed, and likely in your home medicine cabinet. It should be emphatically noted that while they may help acute pain and inflammation, they have significant side effects, especially when given long-term, most notably gastrointestinal bleeding and fluid retention. There are also associated liver problems with most of these drugs. But please do not despair; there are many other drug options available to treat pain. The arsenal of useful prescription drugs for pain management is large – perhaps as many as 200. Add the number of herbal and homeopathic options and the choices become over-whelming (See *Arthritis: The Doctor's Cure & The Aspirin Alternative* by M.W. Loes & David Steinman).

Nerve pain is different from bone and muscle pain. Nerve pain is not usually "inflammatory" or "nociceptive." The characteristic description of "knifelike, sharp, lancinating, lightning bolts" more aptly describes the sensation of nerve pain as opposed to bone pain – "the rusty hinge problem," or muscle pain, "the knotted rope" problem. The treatment for nerve pain focuses on "neuro-modulation," which means that the solution lies in reprograming the messengers that are involved in relaying the pain signals.

Nerve pain is sub-classified as being either **peripheral nerve pain**, or **central nerve pain**. Some authorities assign a third category known as **sympathetically mediated nerve pain** i.e., involving the autonomic nervous system. There are specific transmitters for these nerve pathways – both centrally and peripherally, as the chart below indicates. There are drugs and nutritional supplements that can be brought to bear on each of these mediators.

Neuropeptides	*Hormones*
Glutamate (Primary Neuron)	Serotonin
Substance P (Primary Neuron)	Noradrenalin
NMDA (N-methyl-d-aspartate) (2° Neuron)	Dopamine
AMPA (2° Neuron)	GABA
Endorphins – Beta, enkephalins, dynorphins	Acetylcholine

We know that serotonin and noradrenalin are center-stage players in nerve pain, so it is immensely important to get familiar with the drugs or nutritional supplements that augment the levels or increase the flow of these messengers. Serotonin has become a household word because of its known effect on depression and its crucial role in migraine headaches. There are many prescription drugs that will raise serotonin and some of these are very familiar even to the layperson, especially fluoxetine

(Prozac). Other members of this class include sertraline (Zoloft), paroxetine (Paxil), and citalopram (Celexa). There are also drugs that raise noradrenalin, which is vitally important in restoring balance to the vascular system. Examples of these agents include imipramine (Tofranil), desipramine (Pamelor), and doxepin (Sinequan). These drugs help restore neurovascular tone, rebalance temperature problems, control unwanted vasoconstriction, decrease abnormal sweating, and can lower anxiety as well as control depression.

In other cases, raising dopamine may be important and this can be done with amoxapine (Asendin). Raising dopamine is often helpful in restoring normal musculoskeletal movements. Another pathway that is open to modulation is the GABA (Gamma-aminobutyric acid) pathway. This messenger will aid in raising the pain gate and lowering the irritating effect of peripheral glutamate. Drugs that do this include gabapentin (Neurontin), topiramate (Topamax), and a drug in the pipeline called pregabalon.

Nerve pain may be generated centrally and peripherally and the physician's task is to use drugs that reduce the pain signals. This requires some knowledge and experience.

Mental Emotional (ME Pain)

There is a specialized form of nerve pain called "mental emotional" pain. In the traditional model of medicine, the mind and the body are separate. This is not the case in the energetic model. The brain, after all, is the "seat of the nervous system." When you are sad, confused, and unable to cope, there is real discomfort. There are imbalances that need to be corrected. There are likely cellular communication problems that need to be solved. The same drugs that are used to treat nerve pain are likely the same drugs that your doctor will generally prescribe for depression and anxiety. There may be additional recommendations such as certain nutritional supplements that either boost the battery or speed up the flow of healing energy.

Pain engages our energies. Pain will sap the vitality out of our lives and may go so far as to destroy the innermost self. The Healing Response and the ten principles and laws of healing allow us to approach the management of pain differently. The basis of the approach is energetic – assessing the needs and meeting them. The result can be miraculous. A bleak life can reclaim salubrity. I have seen it. Despair can be tilled under and hope can emerge. Vitality can be nourished and relationships restored. When energy is not moving smoothly, body rhythms are mired down. When one follows the principles and laws of healing, cells can be fed, waste can be washed out, and communication can be enhanced. What results is a process of cleansing negative thoughts, mending wounds, and moving to a better future.

If you are experiencing pain, getting struck and being stuck is more than metaphysical. It can be an energetic coiled snake that is choking you. We must unwind the problem beast, and let the cry come out. When this is done, healing occurs. A balanced life returns. Salubrity is reclaimed.

HEALING WOUNDS & FRACTURES

THE TOPIC OF RAPID WOUND AND FRACTURE HEALING is important to all of us. We get cut and bruised, fall and fracture something. Suddenly, a trip to the emergency room is required. Surgery is sometimes necessary when gallstones clog the bile duct, an appendix acts up, bones are badly broken, or blood vessels threaten to shut down in the heart. A 911 call goes out to the surgeon. The request is "Get me back to normal quickly, please!"

Into the operating room we go. Through the pain and urgency, we look at the surgeon and say: "No lumps, bumps or scars please! No pain please! Will I be able to go home tomorrow?"

Our energies and our fears are narrowly focused on this experience we would rather not be having. We want our health immediately restored and we are depending upon the surgeon to do it.

Wound and fracture healing is of great interest to every one of us. It is also of great importance to the insurance companies who are trying to get us in and out of the hospital as soon as possible.

THE EMPHASIS

Learning how to mount a strong and effective healing response is an effort well worth your time and energy.

THE GOAL

Let's review what is known and then to teach you some simple ways to enhance the healing of your wounds and fractures when it becomes necessary, as no doubt it will.

Pulling a textbook off the shelf from 1986, called *Pathophysiology* by C.M. Porth, it admits that little is known about wound healing and rather pessimistically states the following:

"Science has not found any way to hasten the normal process of wound repair, but there are many factors that impair healing. These include old age, poor oxygen, infection, diabetes, or the presence of cancer." (p124).

In the last decade, the situation has improved, though not as dramatically as one might expect given the rapid progress in science. What progress has been made has not been widely embraced. For example, it is rare that a pre-operative assessment goes beyond the routine measurement of hemoglobin, white blood cells, platelets, liver and kidney function.

The following is a list of statements that are true in regards to wound and fracture healing. They are so general that specific references to support them would be hard to find. It is unlikely that anyone would argue them.

○ The young heal more rapidly than the old.
○ Individuals who are well nourished heal more rapidly than those with poor nutritional status.
○ Patients who do not smoke heal more rapidly than smokers.
○ People who do not drink alcohol heal better than alcoholics.
○ Patients without diabetes heal more rapidly than diabetics.
○ Patients who get out of bed, and begin moving about within 24-48 hours of surgery heal more quickly.
○ Patients who are motivated, and have families depending on them, heal more quickly than those who do not.

The following statements are more specific. There may be a few that would lift an eyebrow if given too emphatically to a medical audience, but there is considerable data to support each of them.

○ Individuals who are not on Non Steroidal Anti-Inflammatory Agents (NSAIDs) heal more rapidly than those that take NSAIDs.

○ Patients who receive adrenal corticosteroids delay acute wound healing.

○ Patients receiving topical proteolytic enzymes heal their burns more quickly.

○ Minerals are important for healing, especially **zinc**, which is required as a co-factor in nearly every biochemical reaction involved in healing. **Sulfur** is very important in that this mineral is part of the structural support for collagen and other connective tissue. **Magnesium** is the crucial mineral for muscle spindle function and normal contractility; its vasodilation action is essential for normal vascular function. **Calcium** is foundational for bone repair. **Boron** is part of the bone matrix and must be present for optimal repair.

○ Branched change amino acids, especially **arginine**, are essential for heal-ing. It stimulates the production of growth hormone that is involved in new tissue growth. **Cysteine** and **glycine** are needed for the synthesis of the mucopolysaccharides by the fibroblast.

○ **Vitamin C** enhances collagen repair and stimulates capillary develop-ment. **Vitamin A** stimulates epithelialization. **Vitamin E** improves the quality and speed of healing by providing antioxidant protection. **Vitamin D** is absolutely essential in building bones. **Vitamin B$_{12}$** is a key nutrient to building blood, especially white blood cells. Lack of **Vitamin K** will retard blood clotting, the first step in wound repair.

○ **Glucosamine Sulfate** is an essential building block for the proteoglycans of cartilage.

○ **Essential Fatty Acids** such as **Docosahexaenoic Acid** (DHA), an omega-3 fatty acid derived from cold-water fish, such as tuna and salmon, is essen-tial in building neuronal membranes.

○ **Oral proteolytic enzymes** assist and help control inflammation by stimu-lating specific immune enhancing events in the human body. They do all of the following: induce optimal amounts of tumor necrosis factor and interleukins, especially interleukin 1-* and interleukin-6, lead to dose-dependent increases in the formation of tumor necrosis factor (TNF-*), reduce edema by enhancing cellular chemotaxis, eliminate extracellular edema, increase cell consuming macrophages, destroy circulating immune complexes, and decrease Transforming Growth Factor (TGF-E) thereby preventing sclerosis, fibrosis, and vulnerable plaque formation.

CLINICAL VIGNETTE #11

Dr. Sara Thompson was a sociology professor at Arizona State University. She was in her late fifties and, overall, she was pretty healthy. She felt she was aging a little faster than she fancied, and sought assistance from a plastic surgeon in getting her wrinkles lifted. She underwent a standard face-lift procedure and the postoperative course seemed normal enough – at first.

Her wounds did not heal as rapidly as anticipated. She expected 7-10 days of discomfort and a good result within 3-6 weeks. But this did not happen. She continued to have a burning, very uncomfortable tingling along her facial suture lines. She returned to the plastic surgeon, who was not very sympathetic. After her first follow-up visit, she decided not to return and she looked elsewhere for help.

She had read something about reflex sympathetic dystrophy on the World Wide Web and someone scared her by suggesting she might have it. She began looking for a place to be evaluated in a different light, and scheduled an appointment at the Arizona Pain Institute at Maricopa Medical Center, the large teaching hospital in Phoenix. Her first visit was about 12 weeks after her facial lift surgery. On exam, she had persistent redness, and exquisite sensitivity along the scar lines. She had an established chronic inflammation with redness, swelling, heat and pain. She was frustrated.

Nothing seemed amiss except that she was taking daily ibuprofen – a lot, about 8 tablets a day of the 200 mg over-the-counter brand, Advil. It helped her pain – a little, but not much. She had continued to take the pills because she thought she was helping the situation because, after all, ibuprofen is an "anti-inflammatory."

She was told by our staff to immediately get off the ibuprofen and to take instead, zinc oxide 30 mg per day, magnesium chloride (slow release) 64 mg tabs, 4 per day, and Vitamin C – 2 grams per day.

She returned in two weeks and she was well on her way to regaining her salubrity, and being healed completely.

THE NSAID CONTROVERSY

"The most popular drugs for arthritis—NSAIDs have been proven to reduce the metabolic capacity of the cartilage, and this could impair articular function in the long run."

> — Pujalte JM, Llavore EP, Ylescupidez FR. Double Blind Clinical
> Evaluation of Glucosamine Sulfate in the basic treatment of
> Osteoarthritis: *Current Medical Research Opinion* in 1980: 7, 110-114

Open wounds, fractured bones, and diseased joints are not likely to improve with long term NSAID use, even if the NSAID used is one of the newer, more selective agents such as rofecoxib (Vioxx) or celecoxib (Celebrex). In fact, there is an increasing opinion that NSAIDs adversely affect the body's balance of prostaglandins, a family of fatty acids involved in the body's inflammatory processes.

The shortsighted view is that while NSAIDs reduce the signs and symptoms of osteoarthritis & rheumatoid arthritis they are making the patients happy only for the short run. They get pain relief. They can get back to their activities of daily living and often, even back to some recreational sports. NSAIDs bring short-term relief to millions of people, but they do not eliminate the underlying disease.

Taking NSAIDs every day, and long-term, does not offer an enticing risk benefit ratio. On average, relief is short-term, and the person taking NSAIDs daily has a six percent chance of ending up in the hospital during any year of chronic therapy. If the individual taking chronic NSAIDs also has or is prone to congestive heart failure, he or she doubles the chance of being hospitalized for shortness of breath due to fluid accumulation.

HAVING SURGERY?
WHAT SHOULD YOU DO?

BEFORE SURGERY, THERE ARE VARIOUS THINGS YOU CAN DO to increase the rate of recovery. If your physician is willing, get a comprehensive nutritional and metabolic assessment. See the Resources section. Pay attention to your stress level the week prior to surgery and keep it low. Get to bed at a regular, scheduled time. Be sure to stay on a balanced diet, higher than usual in leafy green vegetables.

Think Sensibly. Get off aspirin at least three weeks prior to surgery, six if possible. If you have a heart condition, discuss it with your heart doctor. Get off all long-acting NSAIDs, such as piroxicam (Feldene) or oxyprosin (Daypro) a week or two prior to surgery, longer if possible. Try to get off even the intermediate-acting NSAIDs. If you are a little stiff from your arthritis when you do this, take oral proteolytic enzymes as a substitute for the NSAID prior to surgery.

Boost Your Vitamins! Boost Your Minerals! Boost Your Enzymes! Boost Your Hydration! Plenty of clear, healthy water will help your system be ready for the stress of the upcoming surgery.

Think Positive. Go back and review Principle & Law #7. Good healthy thoughts will aid in your recovery.

When your surgery is over and your wound is beginning to heal, get busy quickly moving about as soon as it is safe to do so.

It's not hard to heal quickly and completely. You just have to pay attention to what you know is the right thing to do and then do it. Be sure not to feel sorry for yourself if you are a little uncomfortable. Enviable Health —Salubrity—is right around the corner.

IRRITABLE BOWEL SYMDROME & CHRONIC FATIGUE

IN OCTOBER 2000, I AUTHORED A BOOK called *The Healing Power of Jerusalem Artichoke Fiber* (Freedom Press [www.freedompressonline.com]). The message of the book is that it is very important to have abundant healthy gastrointestinal flora in the small bowel and colon. If these are not present, you will have dysbiosis—abnormal bacterial growth patterns—and frequently, disturbing symptoms are likely to develop: fatigue, weakness, bloating, emotional instability, diarrhea, and constipation.

Jerusalem artichoke is unique in that it contains abundant quantities of inulin, a hugely important prebiotic, which can be extracted from the artichoke and made available as a nutritional substance. This substance will then enhance bowel health by selectively encouraging healthy microflora of the gastrointestinal tract.

In a pain practice, bowel discomfort—yes, pain—is second only to musculoskeletal pain problems. Bowel pain is very uncomfortable. It usually comes and goes in "waves," which is typical of nociceptive visceral pain. The location is often poorly localized and often referred to as the "abyss of the abdomen." There may be low- grade fever or even chilling. Urinary urgency and rectal spasm are not uncommon. Abdominal problems are very real and likely account for much more misery than most of us would like to admit. It is the quiet problem that fuels the over-the-counter antacid market and the frequent patterns of laxative abuse.

It should be apparent that it matters what you eat. It is essential that when you eat, your gut is functioning properly. This is especially true for the tiny cells that line the Peyer's patches (M Cells) on the distal small intestine. There must be a lot of little health helpers working on both sides of the gut membranes. On the outside, in the bowel lumen, are microbiota that help to digest the food and extract the nutrients. The gut bacteria are essential in getting the vitamin content from the foods and presenting them to the membranes. At the membranes are the essential fatty acids and, often, carbohydrate residues. These become part of the essential intracellular communication system. The composition of the membrane includes phosphatidyl serine and nicotinamide adenine dehydrogenase (NADH). It is enzymes working through receptors that make the messages effective. The destination for much of these nutrients will be the intracellular mitochondria, which may make up nearly 70 percent of the intracellular content and are responsible for the generation of energy. When all of this is working effectively, energy will be revved out in abundant quantities and you will be able to reclaim salubrity.

Inulin is arguably the ultimate prebiotic. It may be derived from chicory root (an acid extraction) or from Jerusalem artichoke by water extraction (InuFlora™). This prebiotic brings up quickly and hardily the healthy microbiota of the intestine.

The emphasis here is not to build the case for inulin, but to remind you that bowel health and fatigue are related. There are several major diseases where the overbearing fatigue is arguably more painful than the sensory pain of many musculoskeletal injuries and illnesses. In chronic fatigue syndrome, which usually follows infectious type illnesses, the patient experiences prostrating fatigue that can knock their activities down by over one half. Even rising from bed becomes a daily challenge. Going to work often becomes impossible. The causes of chronic fatigue syndrome have been elusive, but we know many of them are related to gastrointestinal dysfunction, which can be diagnosed by looking in the right place.

Scientists have long suspected that changes in populations of bacteria and other microorganisms that reside in our gastrointestinal tract have wide-ranging effects on human health. Now, an intriguing line of recent research indicates that irritable bowel syndrome may result from such altered populations of microflora in the gastrointestinal tract. In other words, persons with IBS appear to have too many bad disease-causing bugs and not enough good ones. This is a relatively new concept to the medical profession but one that we feel is vital for you to tell your doctor about, because it may help you to finally get over your bout with IBS.

"This is really exciting because it points to the cause of the disease," says Mark Pimentel, M.D., assistant director of the gastrointestinal motility program at Cedars-Sinai Medical Center, Beverly Hills, California, and co-author of a recent study in *The American Journal of Gastroenterology* that linked pathogenic bacterial strains to IBS.[6] "Treatments for irritable bowel syndrome to this point have been directed at symptoms, not any cause."

In their study, Dr. Pimentel and co-investigators found that 78 percent of IBS patients have bacterial overgrowth starting from the colon and making its way into the small intestine. "Once they [the pharmaceutical companies] review this information, they will really wonder what they're doing."

Other researchers have found similar results. In a study at the Department of Surgery, Lund University, Lund University Hospital, Sweden, 60 patients with IBS and a normal colonoscopy or barium enema were randomized into two groups, one receiving a bacterial supplement containing the beneficial species *Lactobacillus plantarum* for four weeks, and another an identical placebo but without the active bacterial culture.[7] Twelve months after the end of the study all patients were asked to complete the same questionnaire regarding their symptomatology as at the start of the study. Flatulence was rapidly and significantly reduced in the test group compared with the placebo group. At the twelve-month follow-up, patients in the test group maintained a better overall gastrointestinal function than control patients.

In a 1998 report in *The Lancet*, it was noted that irritable bowel syndrome might be associated with an abnormal gut flora and with food intolerance (often a sign of altered gastrointestinal bacteria populations).[8] Based on a small study of six female IBS patients and six female controls, these researchers found that IBS symptoms may be associated with alterations in the activity of hydrogen-consuming bacteria.

What does all this mean to you? Simply put, if your gastrointestinal tract is not functioning properly, you are not healthy. Are you striving for salubrity? Presumably, the answer is "yes." Then, address your bowel problems. Try and avoid antibiotics if at all possible. Stay off steroids, unless they are needed for a life-threatening illness. Keep your simple sugars to a minimum. Think seriously about being on a prebiotic and/or a probiotic.

HEADACHES & THE
HEALING RESPONSE

MORE THAN 45 MILLION AMERICANS SUFFER from chronic headaches, 16 to 18 million from migraines, 70 percent of whom are women. Some 12 million persons suffer from daily headaches. It is estimated that almost 70 percent of adults in the United States take a painkiller for a headache at least once a month.

The approach to healing headaches through the principles and laws of healing offers a fresh look at an old problem. Our head is pounding and the hammer can't be found. There are lots of expensive drugs out there, and each new one promises more cures, but often delivers only more disappointment.

CLINICAL VIGNETTE #12

Aaron presented to our office at age 17. He was on seven different prescription drugs and having combined toxicities from many of them. He was totally dysfunctional, could hardly get out of bed, and was suffering continual nausea, fatigue, and depression. He thought his life was over. He was told he had "transformed migraines," which to him meant that he had been transformed into a despairing dummy with no life left to live.

Our approach is always to take away as much medicine as possible from the patient as quickly as possible. While it may seem illogical at first to have just gone ahead and put Aaron on methadone, it was the right decision. This allowed us to control his pain and get him off all the other drugs that were giving him so many problems. His body had become a toxic planet, and we needed to get him clean or, at least, cleaner. We got him off verapamil (Kalan-SR), indomethacin (Indocin), Midrin, sumatriptan (Immitrex), valproic acid (Depakote), amitriptyline (Elavil) and a four times per day hydrocodone/ acetaminophen pill. With this combination, he was consuming four grams per day of liver-kidney damaging acetaminophen.

Aaron's vitality was so suppressed by the host of drugs he was on that as the methadone took effect, it was like he was undergoing a rebirth. As his pain became controlled, his activity went up. He began to sleep better. He was able to eat and drink plenty of water. He was able to communicate with others and he could again feel his body. He began to believe he was going to get well again.

Aaron is still on methadone today (30 milligrams three times per day), but his headaches are under very good control. He takes supplemental magnesium and a multiple vitamin, and was able to return to school. He now attends Northern Arizona University and is an engineering student.

There are individuals who may not make enough of their own endorphins or perhaps they have genetically induced vascular sensitivity. Maybe this is why Aaron got his headaches in the first place. But for Aaron, he has his life back and is living again.

What has happened is that his behavior has become normal and his health is continuing to improve. In time, it is likely that his methadone will be reduced, but that is not the major issue. Naturally, eventually we want to be drug-free, but for some people this may not be realistic.

Even with methadone, Aaron now has a high degree of salubrity—and I do believe that someday soon we will be able to remove the methadone as well.

I wish I could put his picture on the page.

The traditional way to classify headaches is to separate the benign ones from those that are considered malignant and progressively life threatening. Benign headaches are common. They are not a major threat to health. This does not mean that benign headaches do not cause pain or hurt.

Benign headaches may come from the musculoskeletal system—muscles and bones. Or they can come from nerves—central, peripheral, or sympathetic.

If headaches come from muscle, we usually treat them with manual techniques, including massage and acupressure. Structural correction may be necessary and osteopathic manipulation can often accomplish this. Craniosacral therapy is another viable option that can often turn off the headache, especially if accompanied by myofascial release therapy.

We may suggest nutrients that heal and relax muscles such as magnesium, or coenzyme Q_{10}. We might recommend an herb such as feverfew or an herbal combination in tincture form such as ash, aspen and golden rod (**Phytodolor®** from Enzymatic Therapy/PhytoPharmica).

When the headaches come from the nervous system, things are a little more complicated, in that the generators can be either central, as in the brain and spinal cord, or can be coming from the peripheral nerves of the cranial or cervical tissue. There are small peripheral nerves in the facet joints (the small joints in the back of the neck). There are other peripheral nerves around and inside the capsule of the temporal mandibular joint. When these tissues are inflamed or the disc is out of place, there may be severe pain. Aside from nociceptors firing in the joint, there are webs of nerves that innervate the area and can cause cranial or extra-cranial neuralgia. There are also nerve pain generators in the blood vessels giving rise to headaches, especially migraines. The variants of migraine generally have a component of sympathetically mediated pain. This can be addressed though various therapies or procedures. Sympathetic blocks with lidocaine may help and there is recent excitement about the use of botulinum toxin for headaches, including migraine. There are drugs that block the alpha-receptors and drugs that block the calcium channels, which open these pathways to intracellular magnesium.

And then there is 5 hydroxy-tryptophane (5-HTP), a clinically validated natural remedy for vascular headaches (e.g., migraines) that may be able to replace many persons' needs for medical drugs. In *5-HTP: The Natural*

Way to Overcome Depression, Obesity, and Insomnia (Bantam Books 1999), Michael Murray, N.D., says: "For all chronic migraine headache sufferers, I have an important message: Give 5-HTP a try. It works."[9]

There are two types of common headaches: vascular and non-vascular. Vascular headaches are characterized by painful throbbing and pounding. Migraines, for example, are vascular in nature. Nonvascular headaches are characterized by steady pain that feels as if a vise were steadily crushing one's head. Use of 5-HTP is indicated for vascular but not nonvascular headaches.

The prime cause of vascular headaches, especially migraines, is excessive expansion of blood vessels in the head. Besides the brain, the blood vessels also contain serotonin receptors. While in the brain, serotonin affects mood and behavior. In the blood vessels, serotonin causes them to either contract or expand. However, when bodily supplies of serotonin are low, this causes the body's serotonin receptors to become overly reactive. In a sense, the body is attempting to make up for its low serotonin levels by decreasing the threshold number of molecules required to trigger various nerve impulses. This is unhealthy. In such cases, even small amounts of serotonin can cause the blood vessels to suddenly and excessively widen, thus leading to throbbing vascular headaches.

Many factors can precipitate a sudden release of serotonin in the body. Among these are food allergies, histamine releasing foods, such as cheese, chocolate and red wine. Chemicals such as nitrates, nitroglycerin, monosodium glutamate and aspartame (i.e., Equal or NutraSweet) can release histamine, and trigger headaches. Caffeine withdrawal, psychosocial stress, hormonal fluctuations, sleep deprivation, sleep excess, muscular tension, weather changes or even glare and eyestrain from computer monitors can cause severe, seemingly relentless headaches.

USUAL TREATMENT

Raising the body's levels of serotonin helps to decrease the sensitivity of the receptors to the chemical and restore balance. In fact, many prescription drugs for migraine headaches affect the body's serotonin levels. Sumatriptan (Imitrex) activates serotonin receptors in the blood vessels that cause constriction. Methysergide (Sansert) blocks the receptors that cause dilation, thus preventing their uptake of serotonin. Antidepressants classified as selective serotonin re-uptake inhibitors (SSRIs) help keep serotonin levels high. These include the popular drugs Prozac, Paxil, Zoloft, and Celexa.

In 1994, the Food and Drug Administration required Sandoz, the manufacturer of methysergide, to warn users that its long-term use could cause lung and heart fibrosis. Some researchers have observed that chronic use of headache drugs may actually worsen the condition and trigger daily headaches.

5-HTP VS. HEADACHE DRUGS

The beauty of 5-HTP is its absence of side effects and complications, combined with proven clinical efficacy. It is not meant to offer immediate relief, but rather to help prevent recurrent chronic vascular headaches.

At the Headache Unit of the Hospital Valle Hebron, in Barcelona, Spain, use of 600 mg daily of 5-HTP was compared to methysergide.[10] After six months, 71 percent of patients taking 5-HTP and 75 percent of users of the prescription drug experienced at least a 50 percent or greater reduction in frequency or severity of their headaches; thus, the results were statistically equivalent. The users of 5-HTP experienced far fewer side effects. "These results suggest that 5-HTP could be a treatment of choice in the prevention of migraine," report researchers.

At the University of Florence, Italy, when 5-HTP was again compared to methysergide, impressive results were achieved with far lower dosages (200 mg daily).[11, 12]

Many more studies, especially with children's headaches, have demonstrated the clinical efficacy of 5-HTP supplements in alleviation of chronic vascular headaches, especially migraines.[13, 14]

Although the dosage of 5-HTP used in the above detailed studies ranged from 200 to 600 mg, it is often not necessary to take that much. Positive results can be seen in many migraine patients even with very low doses. If you are considering taking 5-HTP for migraine prevention, start at a dosage of 50 mg three times per day. After a couple weeks, if you are not experiencing significant improvement, try increasing the dose to 100 mg three times per day. Progress might be slow at first. Give this regimen at least a two-month trial period due to the fact that beneficially altering the body's serotonin receptors' sensitivity occurs gradually. If headaches persist after two months, consider increasing the dosage of 5-HTP to 150 mg four times per day (three times with meals and once before bedtime). This dosage should be continued indefinitely.

Various 5-HTP products are available at health food stores and natural product supermarkets. You might try **Griffonia 5 HTP** (1-800-497-3742/ www.hbcstore.com) in that much of the research was done on this brand.

EMPHASIS

Normal headaches, called benign, come from bones, muscles and nerves. Vascular headaches, now called migraines, come from the nerves around the blood vessels.

There are variants of both of these types and some patients have both, but as we will see, the treatments tend to be a little different.

IMPORTANT HISTORICAL NOTE

A classification issue regarding benign headaches haunts us. This is because musculoskeletal headaches are currently classified as "tension" headaches, which in English suggests that there are emotional components. When the International Association for the Study of Pain (IASP) selected the word "tension," it was meant to indicate "muscle tension" from the French word "tension" (*pronounced tauntzion*). Muscles develop physiological tension, and this word aptly depicts it in the French language, but the word is a very poor choice for the English speaker and listener.

The other arm of the headache classification system refers to malignant headaches. In this context the word "malignant" refers to headaches that are life threatening. This may refer to cancer-associated headaches, or other progressive headaches resultant from conditions such as glaucoma, subdural hematoma, aneurysm, and multiple sclerosis. It should be noted that cancer of the brain usually does not cause headaches. At least initially, other neurological symptoms such as diplopia (double vision) or dropping objects are more common than pain.

The ten principles and laws of healing can be applied to the evaluation and treatment of headaches. When this is done, some fresh options for their treatment emerge. For example, look at Principle #1, the dead battery problem. There are individuals that just do not have enough juice to get through the day. What they do is rely on artificial stimulants to kick their butts from the time they awake, until it is time to literally crash into the pillow again. The usual butt kickers are adrenaline and caffeine. Adrenaline will eventually burn out your adrenal glands, and caffeine will ruin your sleep patterns, and accelerate the loss of juice from your battery. The result is vascular headaches from the unopposed adrenalin, which causes vasoconstriction, and a meltdown of body serotonin from poor sleep.

If you look at Principles #2 and #3, there are often blockages in energy when people are having headaches. This is why acupuncture often works very well. We also know that massage will help push the discordant energy through. If a headache sufferer is hypothyroid, the headaches will be worse, and correcting the thyroid will help immensely by improving energy flow.

If you do not sleep, various pain protection pathways are disturbed (Principle #4). Headache sufferers are frequently on caffeine-containing analgesics that impair the sleep cycle if they are taken after four p.m. Every patient with headaches needs to be cautioned regarding this.

As for Principles #5 and #6, there is no question that the cells of headache patients are usually very deficient in magnesium. Our routine advice is to have our headache patients take slow-release magnesium chloride: two to six 64 mg tablets per day. It is often amazing how quickly relief will occur with this simple suggestion.

Often when someone has a headache, they begin believing that they will always have a headache. It is very important, according to Principle #7, to believe the talk and then walk it. Usually, there are dietary triggers and behavioral activities that will either bring on or aggravate a headache. Learn to recognize them and change your behavior.

When it comes to sound biodynammic structure, we know that bones and joints need to be protected and constantly rebuilt to be healthy (Principles #8 and #9). If you protect with antioxidants, and build with glucosamine sulfate, methysulfonyl methane (MSM), colloidal minerals and lots of water for cellular matrix, headaches will improve.

Last, but not least (Principle #10), is to heal your attitude, and be connected to your God and universe. If you adopt a playful, prayerful attitude, health will be yours.

There is a lot of hope for those with headaches. It is important to realize that headaches are a form of energetic dysfunction. Most of the time, the X-rays and magnetic resonance scans (MRIs) are negative. There are no brain tumors and there are no blood clots. If the energy can be recharged and the circuits made whole again, the relief will be a welcomed result.

PIONEERS OF THE HEALING RESPONSE

"The man who searches out new trails must first be aware of where man
has gone before him. "
   —Anonymous

WE HAVE AN INTERESTING TASK HERE and that is to recognize and
applaud those pioneers that have laid the foundational principles for The
Healing Response. This is particularly difficult because the healing
response, the healing system, the healing mechanism, the healing—*whatever word you choose*—is not referenced or talked about in any standard
medical text. It is an idea that is usually addressed outside of its holistic
concept. For example, we know about wound healing, as in postoperative
pain and wound closure. There are many books on spiritual healing, the
healing of the mind, and healing the emotional wounds of divorce. But on
the healing response itself? Zip! Struck Out!

In 1987, when Norm Cousins was asked to write the preface for *The
Healer Within*, by Steven Locke M.D., he sadly commented on the following:
   "We are confronted here with one of the great paradoxes of medical science. Less is known and taught about the healing system than about any
of the other internal forces that govern human existence."
   "I tried to find out as much as I could on how the body heals itself—
whether with respect to a cut finger or inflammation of the joints or
stomach disorders or a cold, or a major disease and kept running into a
blank wall."

Perhaps our first applause should go to **Dr. Steven Locke**, who authored *The Healer Within*. He was a main figure behind the field of psychoneuroimmunology (PNI). His findings spearheaded the realization that our brain is literally an apothecary capable of filling a wide array of prescriptions for the body, including pain killers. In 1987, he was chair of the behavioral medicine department at Harvard Pilgrim Health Care and a professor of psychiatry at Harvard Medicine School. The subtitle of his book is *The New Medicine of Mind and Body*. Herein, he reviewed many of the important historical figures as he saw them, and briefly discussed their important accomplishments.

Dr. Barrie Cassileth from the University of Pennsylvania unknowingly became a pioneer, when he authored a controversial article in the New England Journal of Medicine entitled "Psychosocial Correlates of Survival in Advanced Malignant Disease." The article that appeared on June 13, 1985 reported on a series of 359 terminal cancer patients. The alleged opinion of Dr. Cassileth was that he was advocating the position that only the inherent biology of the disease determines the outcome and that psychological, emotional or other factors were largely irrelevant. In typical tabloid fashion, the press picked up this misinterpretation. All positive emotions such as hope, faith, laughter, good spirits, and will to live were ridiculed. Dr. Cassileth was shocked at the sensational news. A disclaiming statement did not stop the tide. The audience was not listening. This prompted Dr. Cassileth along with Norman Cousins, then editor of The Saturday Review, to publish four principles that center on the healing system. Citing evidence from the University of California, Los Angeles, they issued the following joint statement:

1 Emotions and health are closely related.

2 Probably numerous emotional and physical factors influence health and disease.

3 Positive attitudes affect the quality of life even when they cannot influence the physical outcome of disease.

4 Panic, not uncommon when cancer is diagnosed, is in itself destructive, and can interfere with effective treatment.

Dr. Norman Cousins, shortly thereafter, released his story, a bedridden tale of his encounter with the stoic face of medicine: *Anatomy of an Illness*. Now published in four languages, with sales of over two million, he spoke to the common man about his personal struggle fighting with a life-threatening illness. He healed himself with laughter, so he tells you in the popular little book. He watched Laurel & Hardy movies and when he ran out of these, he watched Charlie Chaplin. He said that your beliefs mattered in regards to your health and summed his opinion up with the frequently quoted: *"Belief Creates Biology"* statement.

Dr. Hans Selye a few years earlier, in 1974, published an important text called *Stress without Distress* (New York, New American Library, 1974). Most would attribute to him the concept of The Stress Response, or the General Adaptation Response, both concepts central to any discussion of The Healing Response. The book, which followed two years later, is regarded as the classical text: *The Stress of Life*.

Dr. Herbert Benson, in 1975, authored the acclaimed work: *The Relaxation Response* and as Dr. Steven Locke so eloquently stated in *The Healer Within* when discussing this work: "This book is a mandatory purchase for anyone seriously interested in using the mind to keep the body well. The originator of the Relaxation Response explains it clearly and succinctly."

Dr. Walter B. Cannon wrote a classical paper, which cannot be ignored as a pioneer work: "The Stresses and Strains of Homeostasis" published in the *American Journal of the Medical Sciences*, 189: 2, 1935. Many would consider Walter B. Cannon to be the 20th century scientist who brought into medicine the concept of homeostasis. While acknowledgement is due, it is likely that he relied on the earlier concepts of Rudolf Julius Clausius (1850) to whom we owe the first and second laws of thermodynamics.

It should be additionally noted that the "fight and flight response" is generally attributed to Walter B. Cannon. The classic article is: "The Emergency Function of the Adrenal Medulla in Pain and the Major Emotions," *American Journal of Physiology* 33: (1914) 356-72.

Dr. Rudolf Clausius was certainly not the first to talk about energy. We likely owe that to Isaac Newton or even Copernicus. Both of these ancient philosophers and mathematicians knew about gravity between heavenly bodies, and the potential force of the knock on the head when you were hit by the apple falling from the tree. But it is important to appreciate that it was Clausius who laid out, as foundational principles, the first two laws of thermodynamics:

First Law of Thermodynamics: States that a Property called Energy Exists and is based on the Concept of Work.

Second Law of Thermodynamics: Asserts the Existence of Stable Equilibrium States.

Dr. Walther Nernst is the early 20th century German chemist who formulated the 3rd Law of Thermodynamics (1918):

Third Law of Thermodynamics: Matter Tends Toward Random Motion and Energy Dissipates.

From this concept is derived the need to store energy so that it does not dissipate randomly. This led to the Nernst theorem, which is also known as the battery principle.

Behind these concepts is the idea that individual cells and their interactive membranes that hold electrical potentials are able to store energy and produce work as a result of using that energy.

Dr. Ted J. Kapchuk: When the little book entitled *The Web that Has No Weaver* was first published in 1983, its impact was unassuming and quiet. Its simplicity gradually attracted an ever-growing audience. The work has since emerged as the cornerstone text for both beginning and advanced students of Oriental Medicine. Herein are eloquent explanations of the principles behind yin/yang theory, and the philosophical underpinnings of Chinese diagnosis and treatment. Many of the principles and laws of healing have to do with the unidirectional flow of healing energy, the clearing of stasis, and the protection of the body from adverse influences. We need to appreciate how important this influence is as Eastern medical philosophies are being merged with Western therapies.

Dr. Harry K. Beecher: The first to introduce the idea of the placebo effect, which is a physiological response of the body to a sham (fake, sugar pill) medication. This idea has had a powerful effect on all subsequent research aimed at determining the effectiveness of a drug ("The Powerful Placebo," *J. of the American Medical Association*, 159, 1955, 1602-1606).

Dr. W. R. Hess, a Swiss Nobel Prize winning physiologist, wrote *The Functional Organization of the Diencephalon*, New York, Grune and Stratton, 1957. He was able to show in the cat brain that the fight/flight reaction could be produced by stimulation of a particular area of the hypothalamus and that stimulation of another area in the hypothalamus could produce a relaxation response, which he called the trophotrophic response. It was an energetic – an electrical stimuli – that produced these changes. In demonstrating this principle, a foundational acceptance of brain tissue responses as they relate to behavior was shown.

Dr. Max Wolf (1885-1976) founded the New York Institute of Biological Research. He was the personal physician for many of the famous early actors of the New York Ballet and Theatre. Early on, he recognized the importance of vitamins and enzymes. He is considered by most the father of Systemic Oral Enzyme Therapy and spent most of his life investigating further uses of enzymes to enhance healing, as described in *The Aspirin Alternative* authored by David Steinman and myself. The work of Dr. Wolf was carried further under the late Dr. Karl Ransberger (1925-2001), then president of Mucos Pharma (www.mucos.de). Investigations are continuing worldwide, advancing the therapeutic value of oral proteolytic enzymes in many diseases, especially where fibrosis and sclerosis are involved.

Dr. Candace Pert, in *The Molecules of Emotion,* opened up many doors regarding the idea(s) of cellular communication, especially as they relate to pain. Her pioneering work on the group of messengers, called beta-endorphins, further linked awareness states to physiological stimuli. Her ability to bring science to this area cannot be overstated.

Dr. Moses Gumberg: at the University of Michigan, 1900, derived the first "free radical" from triphenylemethane, which came to mean a relatively unstable molecule with one or more unpaired electrons. **Drs. Friedrich Adolf Paneth and W. Hofeditz** in 1929 discovered the existence of methyl and ethyl free radicals. In 1954, American scientists **Drs. Rebecca Gershman** and **Daniel L. Gilbert** linked the development of retrolental fibroplasia in premature babies to oxygen free radicals. It was perhaps their speculation that "most of the damage to living tissues is the result of oxygen free radicals," that catalyzed the oxidative stress theory of chronic disease. This idea was further expanded and popularized by **D. Harman** in 1956 where he linked aging to the lack of antioxidant protection: *The Journal of Gerontology*, 11:298-300, 1956. "Aging: A theory based on free radical and radiation chemistry." Another milestone was achieved in 1968 when **Drs. J.M. McCord** and **I. Fridovich** discovered a natural antioxidant enzyme in the human body, superoxide dismutase (now referred to as SOD). A popular assumption was that antioxidants must come from the diet, but Drs. McCord and Fridovich were able to show that the body also possesses an internal system, an "on-site police force" that can internally generate antioxidants—SOD. **Dr. Lester Pack** in the 1970's did pioneering work regarding antioxidants and the immune system, focusing on their importance in cancer prevention. More recently, **Dr. Daniel Steinberg**, from the University of California in San Diego, proposed that oxidation—or the combining of oxygen free radicals with other low density lipoproteins (LDL) particles in the blood stream—may be the major cause of plaque formation and clogging of the body's blood vessels. Today, there is little question that antioxidants are crucial for enhancing and maintaining The Healing Response.

There are many schools of thought and tiers of individuals that need to be addressed in any comprehensive research endeavor to further credit the pioneers behind The Healing Response, and the Ten Principles and Laws of Healing. These include the early Greek physicians: Drs. Galen, Hippocrates and even back to mythological figure Asclepias, thought to be the first physician. In all of their early writing, the energies of mind, body and spirit were always working together to reclaim health.

The era of the early German Homeopaths, most notably Samuel Hahnemann, and then the American School, under Dr. Horace Kent and his followers, never ceased searching for concepts to bring ideas of healing into a unified educational system.

The hypnosis movement, most notably Milton H. Erickson, who founded the American Society of Clinical Hypnosis, is a key figure in bringing together the powerful energetic influences of indirect suggestions to enhance health and change dangerous behaviors.

In the last ten to twenty years we have seen significant concepts, research and books by these key individuals that deserve recognition for their efforts in this field of healing: Drs. Norm Shealy's *Creation of Health*, Robert Becker's *Body Electric, Cross Currents*, Larry Dorsey, Kenneth Pellitier, Harold Bloomfield's *Healing Anxiety with Herbs, Making Peace with Your Past*, Michael Murray's *Encyclopedia of Natural Medicine*, Gladys McGarrey's *The Physician as Healer*, Joseph Helm's *Acupuncture Energetics*, Bernie Seagel's *Love, Medicine & Miracles*, Larry Dorsey's *Healing Words*, Andrew Weil's *Spontaneous Healing*, Joseph E. Pizzorno (Editor), Michael T. Murray's *Textbook of Natural Medicine*, and Kenneth Pellitier's *Sound Mind, Sound Body*.

There are surely many others that will fill the web, and weave the fabric toward a more comprehensive understanding of The Healing Response. Help us find these individuals, understand their research, and applaud their efforts. Only with humility and very hard work, will this effort be sustained and become part of our health education.

Disclaimer: Any work in progress will likely leave out, slight, or even totally attribute to the wrong person a word, a concept or even substantial research. Let us all be humble and willing to adjust, correct and when necessary, apologize if possible.

Glossary

THE LANGUAGE OF THE HEALING RESPONSE

WHETHER THE NEW SCIENCE IS CALLED ALTERNATIVE, complementary, integrative, longevity, functional, holistic or wholistic medicine is unimportant. It is the language that counts. The evolving language of the new healing must be spelled out and defined. Various words have been coined within particular disciplines, and even subdivisions. These special words are held even "closer to the chest" to those who coined them, thus making them even harder to handle in any given discussion of the problem.

The power of words is underestimated. Words create reality. He who commands the media commands the message and he who commands the message rules the masses. Words make things happen. They shape the argument. They cause war, quell revolution. Behind words you will find passion, allegiance and loyalty that will define or defile a life's work. We know all too well that a misplaced word—a word overheard that shouldn't have been, or a poorly delivered punch line to a joke—a particular word— can have a major impact on the serenity of the moment. Maybe, it is time that the glossaries were at the beginning of the book instead of the end.

Acetyl-L-carnitine: A "carrier molecule," providing essential fatty acids for mitochondrial energy metabolism. It also assists in removing by-products of this metabolic process.

Active movement: Movement initiated by the patient as opposed to passive movement initiated by someone else, such as a therapist doing gentle, passive stretching to restore range of motion in a joint.

Activin: One of a number of cytokines involved in cell signaling.

Acidophilus: One of the friendly flora of the gastrointestinal tract; it contains many natural antibiotics such as acidophlin, lactophilin, and bacteriocidin.

Acrophase: The time in the circadian cycle when a measured activity reaches its highest (acro) peak.

Adrenergic: Having to do with a branch of chemistry in which various kinds of adrenalin (epinephrine) or stimulating types of neurotransmitters are discussed.

Aerobe: Any of a number of bacteria that require oxygen in the environment to grow and multiply.

Aging: Becoming physiologically older. Most chronic "aging" diseases are mediated by fibrosis and sclerosis.

Alpha-linolenic acid (ALA): The mother of the omega-3 family of fatty acids. It is a specific type of fatty acid essential in membrane stabilization. It is an essential nutrient, meaning humans cannot synthesize it and must obtain it from the their diet. Flaxseed and walnut oils have high concentrations.

Alpha-macroglobulin: A transport protein, when activated—i.e., primed, from the resting slow form to the fast form by utilization of systemic oral enzymes, it can pick up, bind, and transport unwanted metabolic debris out of the area. This process is called phagocytosis and is one of the mechanisms that helps to maintain balance in the system.

Amino acid: Any of a class of organic compounds containing at least one amino group (derived from ammonia) and used as a building block for protein in the human body.

Amplitude: The height of the wave peaks. Most biological activities have peaks and troughs of intensity throughout the day. The "waves" have various cycles and the heights, depths, and frequencies define the physiology.

Anaerobe: Any of a number of bacteria that do not need oxygen to survive, but thrive on food in a substrate, independent of oxygen.

Analgesic: Pain relief medication.

Angiogenesis: Formation of new blood vessels. Many tumors spread rapidly because of angiogenesis. Angiogenesis is likely caused, in part, by excessive secretion of TGF-β (Transforming Growth Factor, β Subunit).

Antibody: Protein molecule produced by the immune system's B lymphocyte cells as a primary immune defense. These combine with antigens to disable foreign pathogens.

Antigen: Substances that stimulate the body's production of antibodies.

Antioxidant: Substance that scavenges free radicals and prevents oxidation of bodily tissues and cells.

Arachidonic acid (AA): A type of prostaglandin found almost entirely in animal foods (along with saturated fat), which can increase the body's inflammation levels.

Arthralgia: Pain in joints. There is no noticeable inflammation. This means when a physician examines the joint, there is no redness, swelling or heat objectively present. This does not mean that it does not hurt. Arthralgias are common in lupus erythematosus and fibromyalgia.

Arthritis: Inflammation of joints. There is redness, swelling, heat. This is common in rheumatoid arthritis, though not so common in osteoarthritis. In osteoarthritis, there may just be cracking, popping, clicking, or just plain old disabling stiffness. There are more than 100 types of arthritis— the most common types being osteoarthritis (also called degenerative arthritis), rheumatoid arthritis and gout.

Articular cartilage: Cushioned, watery, highly slick cartilage in the area of the joints at ends of bones composed of glucosamine sulfate, chondroitin, proteoglycans and collagen.

Autocrine: Indicates that there is a feedback loop that stimulates further synthesis of the substance. TGF-β is an autocrine cytokine meaning that once levels are elevated, TGF-β stimulates its own synthesis.

Auto-antibodies: Non specific antibodies made by B lymphocytes, usually against a viral or bacterial intruder that cross-reacts with otherwise normal tissue, which it begins seeking to destroy. In rheumatic heart disease streptococcus, such antibodies can sometimes react against a person's heart valves. In rheumatoid arthritis auto-antibodies destroy joint tissue; and in lupus erythematosus the damage is directed against the kidneys. This cross-reaction causes complexes of circulating C-reactive proteins to increase, and sedimentation rates to rise

Auto-immune: A process by which auto-antibodies are made and the body's immune system turns on or attacks the body's own tissues as in rheumatoid arthritis, lupus erythematosis, scleroderma, dermatomyositis, and even some types of thyroid disease.

Ayurveda: The ancient healing system of India that perceives health as a reflection of the proper balance of life forces within an individual

Bacteria: Microscopic one-celled organisms that have their own genome inside their cellular mitochondria.

Bacteriocidal: Used to refer to antibiotics that kill bacteria directly.

Bacteriostatic: Antibiotics that kill bacteria indirectly by interfering with cell wall synthesis or other aspects of metabolism necessary for growth.

Bioflavonoids: A group of water-soluble compounds that, like vitamins, play a crucial role in countering oxidative stress. These substances were once known as "vitamin P" but not recognized as crucial cellular molecules that have powerful antioxidant properties. They are closely related to vitamin C (ascorbic acid) and are usually yellow in color. They also help to maintain the structural support of many tissues, including collagen.

Blood-brain barrier: Protective layer of cells separating the brain tissues from all other tissues. This barrier precludes many molecules, drugs and other substances from entering the central nervous system. It protects both ways, in that when drugs or substances get into the central nervous system, they also have trouble leaving.

Bone morphogenic proteins: A group of cell messengers, including activin, that signal specific needs to an ever-changing organism.

Bone marrow: Soft, vascular tissue in the cavities of bones where blood cells are formed.

Circadian Acrophase for Peak Performance (CAPP): The point of the body's most profound physiology, for example, the capacity to metabolize ingested alcohol peaks at nine p.m.

Cartilage: Firm, white-blue substance at the ends of bones, which is highly water-dependent, and has no blood vessels. Acts as body's shock absorber.

Cholesterol: A complex molecule used to make steroids. It is the precursor for estrogen, progesterone, pregnenolone and testosterone. It is an essential component of cell membranes. There are various types of cholesterol: high-density lipoprotein (HDL) cholesterol and low-density lipoprotein (LDL) cholesterol. Oxidized LDL causes atherosclerosis. High levels of HDLs help to prevent heart disease.

Cell matrix: The fluid within the cells. There can be rather high electrical gradients between the inside and the outside of cells that make up the biogenic potential—the electromotive force.

Chemical mediator: A molecular biological response activated by a stimulus to meet a physiological need. The need is usually not disease specific. Cytokines are a class of mediators that have been classified and are being intensively studied in an effort to better understand disease.

Chondrocytes: The cells in joints that produce the substances that make up cartilage.

Circadian: "About a day." In humans, the circadian rhythm is a little more than twenty-four hours. Even without outside signals, such as light, food, and activity, this clock would run with amazing precision.

Circulating immune complex (CIC): A glob of antibodies and antigens with other tissue matter formed during inflammatory and auto-immune diseases such as rheumatoid arthritis, and deposited in the body's tissues, causing intense inflammation.

Carotenoids: Plant pigments that usually act as reducing agents and protect against oxidative stress.

Collagen: Substance that makes up the body's connective tissues. Collagen gives cartilage its "spring." The collagen found in joints is called Collagen Type II.

Corticosteroid: Powerful steroid medication that reduces inflammation. Complications include damage to heart, bone, and immune systems. These agents inhibit the production of prostaglandins and white blood cells.

Crepitus: The crackling sound that joints sometimes make with movement, usually indicating surface irregularities of the cartilage.

Cyst: Sac of fluid that forms in bone as cartilage is worn away.

Cytochrome: Area in the cell where metabolism occurs. An example would be the p450 system in the liver, responsible for the metabolism of many drugs.

Cytokine: Various cellular mediators that signal various physiological processes.

Cytoplasm: Watery material inside a cell that surrounds the nucleus. Mitochondria and other important cellular machinery are in the cytoplasm.

Diaita: The Greek concept of diet, but much more expansive in ancient meaning than usually interpreted by the modern word as used by Western medicine. Diaita was meant to refer to a person's entire mode of living—i.e. the relationship between rest and exercise, between sleep and wakefulness, and patterns involving hygiene, sexual practices, and even excretion habits.

Diathesis: Predisposition. Something in the patient's history or environment that will predispose them to a particular kind of problem.

Diadzein: An isoflavone found in food such as soy.

Docosahexaenoic Acid (DHA): An essential fatty acid and member of the omega-3 fatty acid family, derived from cold-water fish such as tuna and salmon, and an essential structural building block for neuronal membranes.

Dosha: Literally means, "that which causes decay," but in Ayurveda refers to the three forces of life: wind, fire, and water.

Duodenal ulcer: A sore in the mucous membrane, located in the first portion of the small intestine.

Dyschronogen: A drug or other influence that has a negative effect on circadian rhythms.

Eicosapentaenoic Acid (EPA): Part of the omega-3 fatty acid group that up-regulates prostaglandin-3 (PGE-3) and down-regulates inflammatory reactions caused by prostaglandin-2 (PGE-2).

Eicosanoids: Humeral factors which contribute to cellular metabolism.

Electromotive force: Most aptly applied in electrical engineering, but in a very real sense, human physiology is directed by its electromotive force, and perhaps, is a preferred, although poorly accepted, term that could embody the idea of "vital force" or "life essence."

Endorphins: A group of protein molecules—beta-endorphin, enkephalins, and dynorphins—that are known for their ability to down-regulate pain signals.

Energy: An unseen force. You see the effects of energy, but not the actual thing. Energy is defined by various equations in physics, the most recognizable being E= mass times the speed of light squared (MC^2), where it relates potential energy to mass. Energy is also described by what is known as quantum mechanics where there is a relationship between mass and wavelength. Of interest is that Einstein's Nobel prize was not for his theory of relativity, but for proving that light has mass—i.e., that it can respond to a gravitational force.

Entrainment: The ability of an activity to synchronize body rhythms, as is reported in deep breathing exercises and various types of yoga.

Entropy: Positive entropy refers to a high state of disorganization whereas negative entropy refers to a higher state of organization.

Enzymes: Large protein molecules that work in a lock and key manner and that embrace, bring together, or separate other molecules to facilitate chemical reactions.

Epidermal Growth Factor: See growth factors.

Excipients: Those extra ingredients in products that serve as lubricants, disintegrants, binders, adsorbents, and glidants. Magnesium stearate is a lubricant; stearic acid is a lubricant and binder; colloidal silicon dioxide is an adsorbent and glidant; cellulose gum is a super-disintegrant; microcrystalline cellulose is a diluent, absorbent, and lubricant; vanillin is a sweetener to mask the odor of other ingredients; titanium dioxide is used to give a white color to the materials.

Extracellular matrix: The fluid "sea medium" between cells that makes up the continuous fluid layer between all cells.

Fascia: A band or sheath of connective tissue covering, supporting, or connecting the muscles or internal organs of the body.

Fatty acid: A group of essential molecular building blocks for such vital structures as membranes, myelin, axons, and brain cells.

Fibronectin: See growth factors

Fibrosis: The process of laying down extra fibrous tissue around organs—connecting tissue that the body does not need (e.g., kidney or liver fibrosis). Fibrosis is also seen as leathering, wrinkling and elastosis (loss of skin elasticity), which are all signs of these processes that involve the skin.

Flatulence: Gas produced by the gastrointestinal tract. When it comes down through the anus, it is called flatulence, but when it comes up from the stomach, it is usually referred to as belching or eructation.

Fructooligosaccharides (FOS): Complex sugar molecules containing fructose and chains of glycogen. They are non-absorbable unless broken down. FOS can act as food to friendly flora of the gastrointestinal tract.

Free radical: Substance or molecular fragment with one or more unpaired electrons that is highly reactive, stripping and damaging other cells in a process called oxidation, as it searches for an electron match.

Functional food: A food that enhances a particular biological function. Among members of The Institute of Functional Medicine (of which I am one), the word "functional" has become a cornerstone concept for anything that improves the dysfunction or early symptoms of an illness. The idea is that illness (dys-ease) will start with symptoms that have their basis in potentially reversible biochemical lesions and that, if identified early on, the patient will more readily regain salubrity—this can occur by supplying the functional foods or conditional nutrients required to effect the reversal of the dysfunction.

Fungi: A group of spore-forming organisms that, when allowed to grow, compete with normal flora and can seriously compromise homeostasis.

Gamma-linolenic acid (GLA): A precursor of the omega-6 fatty acids, essential for structural integrity of neuronal membranes.

Genistein: An isoflavone found in foods such as soy.

Glucosamine sulfate: An amino sugar essential for the structure of cartilage and other connective tissues. Natural glucosamine sulfate is harvested from marine shells. A specific form of glucosamine sulfate is used as an osteoarthritis-healing agent. Glucosamine sulfate is one salt of glucosamine, and glucosamine hydrochloride (HCl) is another. The preferred agent for arthritis and healing cartilage is glucosamine sulfate.

Gluten: A protein in wheat, barley, and rye. When not digested properly, residue peptides can cause allergic and autoimmune responses, as seen in celiac sprue, some cases of regional enteritis, and leaky gut syndrome.

Glycosaminoglycans: A group of polysaccharides, which are responsible for water retention in cartilage. Glycosaminoglycans are the building blocks of proteoglycans.

Gout: Painful inflammation of joints, characterized by an excess of uric acid in the blood, which leads to crystalline deposits in the small joints. The joint most commonly affected is the first metatarsal, the large joint of the big toe.

Growth factors: Chemicals that stimulate cell division and regeneration. When secreted in normal (small) amounts, they are essential to tissue. When secreted in excess, they play an important role in causing fibrosis, sclerosis, and widespread degeneration. The major growth factors are: transforming growth factor-beta (TGF-β); insulin like growth factor (IGF); epidermal growth factor (EGF); platelet derived growth factor (PDGF); and fibronectin. We know more about TGF-β because of research concerning proteolytic enzymes (Wobenzym®N) that shows they normalize the body's production of TGF-β, lessening fibrosis, sclerosis, and the presence of adhesion molecules. That is why Wobenzym®N has attracted such attention as an anti-aging tool.

Health Maintenance Organization (HMO): Organization that delivers medical services to pre-selected caregivers at a fixed price on a prepaid basis.

Herb: A plant valued for its medicinal properties.

Histamine: Derived from the amino acid histidine, histamines are released particularly by mast cells during allergic reactions. They cause dilation, inflammation, and blood vessel permeability.

Holmes-Rahe Social Readjustment Scale: In this test, 43 items are scored and given a numerical value. If your sum is over 300, you have an 80 percent chance of becoming seriously ill in the next year. You can use the items below, checking off which apply, to assess your own risk of illness.

Potential Life Stress	Value
Death of a spouse	100
Divorce	73
Marital Separation	65
Jail Term	63
Death of a family member	63
Personal Injury/Illness	53
Marriage	50
Fired from Work	47
Marital Reconciliation	45
Retirement	45
Changes in family member's health	44
Pregnancy	40
Sex Difficulties	39
Addition to Family	39
Business Readjustment	39
Changes in Financial Status	38
Death of a Close Friend	37
Change to Different Line of Work	36
Mortgage or Loan over $10,000	31
Foreclosure of Mortgage or Loan	30
Change in Work Responsibilities	29
Son or Daughter Leaving Home	29
Trouble With In-laws	29
Outstanding Personal Achievement	28
Spouse Begins or Stops Work	26
Starting or Finishing School	26
Revision of Personal Habits	24

Trouble With Boss	23
Change in Work Hours, Conditions	20
Change in Residence	20
Change in Schools	20
Change in Recreational Habits	19
Change in Church Activities	19
Change in Social Activities	18
Mortgage or Loan Under $10,000	17
Change in Sleeping Habits	16
Change in Number of Family Gatherings	15
Change in Eating Habits	15
Vacation	13
Christmas Season	12
Minor Violation of the Law	11

Homeodynamics: In some academic or philosophical circles, homeodynamics is the preferred term instead of homeostasis. Homeodynamics emphasizes that there is continued "balanced movement." The body is never static.

Homeostasis: Meaning balance, the body must be free of stasis and in harmony to attain homeostasis. In fact, it should not surprise you that the literal meaning of the word poisoned is "loss of balance." Lack of homeostasis causes excessive secretion of growth factors and excessive inflammation.

Homocysteine: An amino acid found in blood that directly correlates with risk of stroke, dementia, Alzheimer's disease, and myocardial infarction. Fortunately, vitamin B_{12} will directly lower the homocysteine level, but if vitamin B_{12} is normal and homocysteine is high, it is likely that the body's stores of vitamin B_{12} are functionally low or ineffective.

Hyperbaric oxygen: The administration of highly concentrated oxygen under pressure to promote healing in non-healing wounds. Use of hyperbaric oxygen has found use in wound healing and multiple sclerosis therapy. It seems to provide a better milieu for myelin repair and down-regulates the hyperreactive immune system seen in multiple sclerosis. (See brainrecovery.com)

Immune complexes: Conglomerates of immune cells usually made up of an antibody-antigen complex, but may be a mass of other foreign material with immune reactive cells attached.

Inflammation: A physiological reaction characterized by redness, swelling, heat and pain. There is also loss of function. In acute inflammation, the process is rapid and usually humerally mediated—in other words, there is a rapid blood response with platelets, white blood cells (granulocytes and B lymphocytes), and a glandular response with secretions of hydrocortisone and epinephrine by the adrenals.

Interleukin-1 (IL-1): The cytokine that prominently regulates fever in the inflammatory process. When high, IL-1 has been implicated in the loss of appetite, depression, lethargy and pain. Recent research suggests that IL-1 plays a role in promoting atherosclerosis, endometriosis, and osteoporosis.

Intermittent reinforcement: In contrast to scheduled or timed reinforcement, with intermittent reinforcement a reward is given at unpredictable times. This type of reinforcement is associated with considerable stress, in that one does not know when they will be appreciated or rewarded.

Isoflavones: Molecules found in some foods, especially soy, that have a potential to influence human chemistry by virtue of their similarity to the sex hormone, estrogen.

Isometrics: A form of exercise in which immovable pressure is applied, such as pressing hands against each other, neck against hand, or pushing into a wall.

Law of simplicity: As applied to human physiology, biological reactions get simpler as the patient gets sicker. The physiology of the patient begins to rely on the very core of life—like breathing and heartbeat. All of the accessory systems of defense have been destroyed or used up.

Leaky gut syndrome: A condition wherein the membranes of the gut are highly permeable, allowing large antigenic molecules to pass into the systemic circulation and cause disease. There are cracks in the gastrointestinal membrane, especially between cells, allowing leakage of larger molecules.

Leukotrienes: Lipids produced by white blood cells in an immune response to antigens that contribute to allergic asthma and inflammatory reactions.

Ligament: Band of strong connective tissue that connects bones and holds organs in place.

Lignans: Plant pigments found in many foods such as whole rye and flax seeds, lignans release chemicals that influence human chemistry and appear to reduce risk of cancer spread.

Lipids: All fatty molecules, which are insoluble in water.

Longevity: The science of aging—and obtaining a long life.

Medicine: From the Latin word "medico" meaning "I drug."

Melatonin: A derivative of serotonin that acts as an antioxidant and message-carrying molecule and which activates and regulates the dark/sleep cycle of humans. The peak of melatonin level in the blood is at about 3:00 AM, and is one of the sharpest and narrowest of all the body's circadian cycles.

Miasmata: Noxious vapors generated from the bowels of the earth. Often thought to be the cause of various illnesses in the Middle Ages.

Mitochondria: Cigar-shaped compartments inside cells where most of the energy metabolism takes place. It is here where phosphate bonds are generated and cleaved. Mitochondria resemble bacteria in many ways in that they have their own genome.

Neurotransmitter: Refers to a class of mediators that influence mood, alertness and sensation. These include serotonin, noradrenalin, acetylcholine, dopamine, endorphins, as well as substance P.

Nitric oxide: Declared molecule of the year in 1992 by *Science* magazine, nitric oxide is known to vasodilate and improve peripheral circulation. It is also known to be involved in the modulation of pain signals. It relaxes the muscles in the vessel walls and helps promote blood flow to the areas of the heart, but also to other areas of the body. Nitric oxide has been found in the brain and may be a very important molecule in the storage of memory. Nitric oxide is synthesized from the amino acid arginine and is likely directly involved in many biological processes. Its role in the onset of juvenile diabetes is under scientific exploration.

Nonsteroidal Anti-Inflammatory Agents (NSAIDs): These are drugs, such as aspirin, that act to inhibit the cyclo-oxygenase (COX) system. Specifically, they inhibit two isoforms of the enzymes—COX-1 or COX-2. Because most of the NSAIDs inhibit both, they upset bodily homeostasis, since we rely on COX-1 to keep the stomach safe and maintain its mucosal lining integrity. There are newer NSAIDs that selectively inhibit COX-2 such as celecoxib (Celebrex) and rofecoxib (Vioxx). These are safer, but not completely safe.

Opioid: An "opiate" refers to morphine, or codeine specifically derived from the poppy plant, but the term "opioid" is broader and includes semi-synthetics such as ocycodone (Percodan), hydrocodone (Vicodin) and synthetic drugs such as meperidine (Demerol), methadone (Dolophine) and fentanyl (Duragesic), that act on the central pain receptors.

Osteoarthritis: The "wear and tear" or biomechanical form of arthritis, as opposed to rheumatoid arthritis, which is an auto-immune disease.

Osteophytes: Mineralized outgrowths of bone in damaged cartilage areas.

Passive movement: Movement initiated or aided by another person.

Phase Shift: A resetting of the acrophase to either earlier or later.

Pluripotentiality: The sum of various of the body's healing responses coming together to restore health.

Precipitating event: Any event, usually a very mild trigger that sets an illness into motion.

Primed: A cell is primed when it is "ready to go." This is another term for "activated." A quiescent cell is "non-primed" and resting. There are lots of synonyms or metaphors for cells that are either in the fight or on the sidelines.

Probiotic: A dietary supplement that contains bacteria grown outside the body and then is ingested by the person to assist the further development of beneficial bacteria in the colon—usually refers to acidophilus, lactobacillus and bifidobacteria.

Prostaglandins: Hormone-like fatty acid substances that influence the body's inflammation levels, temperature, muscular contractions, and many other functions. As with cholesterol, health specialists classify these substances as either "good" prostaglandins or "bad" prostaglandins. We need both, but it is still a useful classification.

Prostanoids: Substances made by every living cell in response to stress. They are signal molecules. This word refers to a class of molecules known as prostaglandins.

Protein: Composed of long chains of amino acids and constituting much of the mass of living organisms.

Proteoglycans: Mortar-like substances made from protein and sugar that are the building blocks of cartilage.

Protozoa: Small, parasitic organisms that can cause disease. Technically not bacteria because of their structure, but fully capable of major illness (i.e. syphilis).

Reactive Oxygen Species (ROS): Another name for free radicals—molecules missing an electron and on a suicide mission to find one. Hopefully, if the body is healthy, there will be adequate antioxidants available to fill the need so that the ROS does not have to take it from a membrane or an essential nucleotide.

Recruitment: The ability of a cell or system to bring up help. Various cells, even of a different type, are called upon to help out with the problem.

Reinforcement: When the system or subsystem is failing, there may have to be reinforcements; however, their ability to be there and to help will depend on the health of the system.

Remedy: The homeopathic prescription that contains usually a mineral or herb in a diluted, energized form.

Rheumatoid arthritis: The autoimmune form of arthritis.

Rhythm: Biological rhythm is the clockwork of your physiology. When it is tuned, you tend to feel better. When it is out of synch, you tend to have problem. These are examples of a person who is in rhythm:

○ I wake up in the morning without an alarm clock.

○ I feel well rested after a night's sleep.

○ I spend time each day in quiet reflection, prayer, or relaxation.

○ I spend most of the day on my feet.

○ I walk briskly for thirty minutes or more every day.

○ I engage in sports activities.

○ I go to bed and wake up at about the same time each day.

○ On weekends, I get up at about the same time as on weekdays.

○ I get fresh air and sunshine.

○ I eat leisurely, enjoying my meals.

○ I engage in strenuous work.

Sclerosis: The process of laying down "hardening materials" such as calcium to form hard plaques as in coronary artery disease (atherosclerosis).

Serotonin: A neurotransmitter that is very abundant in the gastrointestinal tract and in the brain. Its level in the blood is typically higher at night and is associated with sleep. Its modulation is the target of many drugs used to treat depression.

Slow Acting Drug in Osteoarthritis: Specific term applied to glucosamine sulfate by the International League Against Rheumatism.

Statistics: The rendering of physiology to numbers as groups, but not as singular individual physiology. There was never a statistical human. An unknown sage referred to statistics as "people with tears removed."

Steroids: There are two major classes of corticosteroids, commonly called "steroids." Those derived from cortisone are known as anti-inflammatory steroids and are very potent anti-inflammatory agents, but they are known to have multiple long-term, dangerous side effects. When given for prolonged periods in high doses, these will cause overgrowth of opportunistic infections such as yeast, most notably candida. The other class of steroids is known as anabolic steroids, often used by athletes to bulk up.

Sulfate: Derived from sulfuric acid, sulfates are a nutrient for the body's joint matrix and many other tissues.

Substance P: A substance in the blood known to produce pain and cause vasodilatation. It is the algesic (pain-causing) substance of the secondary pain receptors. There are topical creams on the market such as acyclovir (Zovirax), which direct its action to decreasing this substance in painful tissue.

Symbiosis: The mutual and harmonious living together of various bacteria.

Synchronous: Directed, harmonious. When the term refers to light, it means that the wavelengths are all directed in the same direction.

Synovial fluid: A clear, viscous, lubricating fluid found in joints.

Synovial membrane (also known as synovium): The soft encapsulating material surrounding the joint that allows nutrients, toxins and other liquids to pass in or out.

T-Helper cells: The T-lymphocytes are the major cell defense for cell-to-cell mediated immunity, especially when it comes to dealing with viruses and cancer. There are various subdivisions of T—cells called CD—from the "Center for Disease" classification system. There are nearly 200 CD cells. T-cells work with each other to mount a defense.

Tendons: White, fibrous cord or band that connects muscles to bones.

Thromboxane: Substance formed in blood platelets, which causes clotting.

Transforming growth factor-beta (TGF-β): This substance is likely the master switch for almost all tissue repairs. Virtually every cell in the body—including epithelial, endothelial, hematopoietic, neuronal and connective tissue cells—produce TGF-β and have receptors to which it may attach. Although originally discovered as a tumor growth factor, TGF-β is considered a multifunctional cytokine, perhaps the major messenger protein in the body. It initiates and turns off tissue repair, but if left on too long, as often happens with aging, it can result in tissue overgrowth and hardening of tissues resulting in atherosclerosis, cancer, and metastasis of cancer cells, including the accelerated formation of new blood vessels needed for tumor growth (a process called angiogenesis). Growth factors are needed in childhood, but in adulthood, although required, often become over-expressed. This is where systemic oral enzymes help, as they normalize production of TGF-β.

Triglycerides: These are fatty acids held together by other small molecules, usually a glycerol chain.

Tryptophane: An amino acid from which serotonin and melatonin are formed.

Tumor necrosis factor (TNF): A very important cytokine that can kill cancer cells and hence has been the subject of developing pharmacology.

Ultradian: Meaning "less than a day," for example, rhythms that cycle many times a day—such as our breathing which occurs approximately sixteen times every minute.

Yin-yang: The core balance of energy in Traditional Chinese Medicine. Yin-yang refers to passive (yin) and active (yang) and female (yin) and male (yang), and many other polar concepts that have relative strengths within each individual. In fairness, a simple definition cannot be given.

Xenobiotic: An invader foreign to the body as in some bacteria, fungi, viruses, or protozoa.

Zeitergeber: From the German (*zeit* for time and *geber* for giver), this is an influence such as light, activity, food, or drugs that tends to change or reinforce the body's circadian rhythms.

Resources

WHERE TO FIND HELP

TO LOCATE A HEALTH PRACTITIONER who is aware of *The Healing Response* and who emphasizes a natural healing program utilizing concepts reported in this book contact the following groups:

American Association of Naturopathic Physicians
2366 Eastlake Avenue, Suite 322
Seattle, WA 98102, (206) 323-7610

American Chiropractic Association
1701 Clarendon Boulevard
Arlington, VA 22209, (703) 276-8800

American College of Advancement of Medicine
23121 Verdugo Drive, Suite 204
Laguna Hills, CA 92653, (714) 583-7666

American Academy of Medical Acupuncture
4929 Wilshire Boulevard, Suite 428
Los Angeles, CA 90010, (323) 937-5514
Web Site: www.medicalacupuncture.org

American Academy of Orthopedic Medicine
P.O. Box 4997
Buena Vista, CO 81211, (800) 992-2063
Web Site: www.aaomed.org

American Academy of Pain Management
13947 Mono Way, #A
Sonora, CA 95370, (209) 533-9744
Web Site: www.aapainmanage.org

American Academy of Pain Medicine
& American Chronic Pain Association
4700 West Lake Avenue
Glenview, IL 60025-1485, (847) 375-4731
Facsimile: (847) 375-6331
Web Site: www.painmed.org

American Association of Orthopedic Medicine
30897 C.R. 356-3
P.O. Box 4997
Buena Vista, CO 81211, (800) 992-2063

The American College of Rheumatology
1800 Century Place, Suite 250
Atlanta, GA 30345, (404) 633-3777
Facsimile: (404) 633-1870
e-mail: acr@rheumatology.org
Web Site: www.rheumatology.org

American Pain Society
4700 West Lake Avenue
Glenview, IL 98105, (847) 375-4715
Web Site: www.ampainsoc.org

Arizona Institute of Minimally Invasive Spine Care
1635 E. Myrtle Ave
Phoenix, AZ 85020, (602) 216-6099

The Arizona Pain Institute
Education & Research
14861 N. Cave Creek Road
Phoenix, AZ 85032, (602) 992-1486, fax: (602) 992-6604
Web Site: www.arizonapaininstitute.com

Arthritis Foundation
1330 W. Peachtree
Atlanta, GA 30309, (404) 872-7100 or (800) 283-7800
Web Site: www.arthritis.org

Institute of Functional Medicine

5800 Soundview Drive
P.O. Box 1729
Gig Harbor, WA 98335, (800) 228-0622
Web Site: www.fxmed.com

International Pain Foundation

909 NE 43rd Street, Suite 306
Seattle, WA 98105, (206) 547-2157

The National Pain Foundation

2616 South Milwaukee Street
Denver, CO 80210, (303) 692-8414
e-mail: TNPF@aol.com
Web Site: www.TNPF.org

NUTRIENT & IMMUNOLOGICAL TESTING

Amino Acids and Fatty Acids

Metametrix
4855 Peachtree Ind. Blvd.
Norcross, GA 30092, (800) 221-4640

B Complex

Spectracell Labs, (800) 227-5227
B vitamin tests & determination of functional levels.

Immunological Testing

Immuno Labs, Inc.
1620 West Oakland Park Boulevard, Suite 300
Fort Lauderdale, FL 33311, (800) 231-9197

Minerals

Doctor's Data, (800) 323-2784

Great Smokies Diagnostic Laboratories

63 Zillicoa St. Ashville, NC, 28801-1074
(800) 522-4762
Facsimile: (828) 252-9303
e-mail: cs@gsdl.com
Web Site: www.gsdl.com

Vitamin, Antioxidants, and CoenzymeQ Tests

Pantox, (888) 726-8698

SUBSCRIBE TO **THE DOCTORS' PRESCRIPTION FOR HEALTHY LIVING**

The Doctors' Prescription for Healthy Living is a newsletter dedicated to informing consumers about the latest information in health trends and products that make sense. Its vision is health education. The goal is to have various physicians and health educators look at new products and trends and discuss them in an easy to read format that will excite you and help you improve your health.

The editor of **The Doctors' Prescription for Healthy Living** is David Steinman who has co-authored several books with Dr. Michael Loes, as well as writing hundreds of professional articles and books on his own prior to working in tandem with Dr. Loes on multiple projects. Two of David Steinman's most popular books are **The Safe Shopper's Bible** and **The Breast Cancer Prevention Program**, available on Amazon.com.

The newsletter makes brand name recommendations after carefully researching available products, and also teaches consumers about medically validated pathways of natural healing for conditions such as depression, enlarged prostate, menopausal symptoms, high blood pressure and cholesterol, diabetes, obesity, and other common health problems.

It's a great newsletter that makes sense. We believe it should be in every family's home. Cost is only $29.95 for 12 issues. An introductory package is available where several books of your choice will be included with the initial subscription. View the website: freedompressonline.com Send your check or money order (no cash) to Freedom Press, 1801 Chart Trail, Topanga, CA 90290 or follow directions on the Web Site. You may also call their toll-free number at 1-800-959-9797 for further information.

About the Author

MICHAEL LOES, M.D., M.D.(H.)

MICHAEL W. LOES M.D., M.D.(H), completed medical school at the University of Minnesota, followed by a fellowship in clinical pharmacology. His residency training was in Internal Medicine at the University of Arizona in Tucson.

Dr. Loes is certified by boards or qualifying exams in Internal Medicine, Pain Medicine, Pain Management, Alcohol and Chemical Dependency, Acupuncture, Clinical Hypnosis, Homeopathy, and Disability Medicine. He is on the Board of Directors for the National Pain Foundation and Arizona Teen Challenge. An assistant professor at the University of Arizona, he is currently Director of the Arizona Pain Institute in Phoenix. He is consultant to Southwest Pain Management and Southwestern Center for Pain and the Arizona Institute for Minimally Invasive Spine Care. He has co-authored *Arthritis: The Doctors' Cure; The Non-drug European Secret to Healing Sports Injuries Naturally; The Aspirin Alternative;* and *The Healing Power of Jerusalem Artichoke Fiber.* All of these books have their roots in traditional medicine, but their heart in functional integrative medicine

Dr. Loes has been involved in pain research for nearly 20 years and has authored numerous professional articles. Writing and speaking have always been a primary thrust of Dr. Loes's endeavors, having started at age eighteen, when he was the senior editor of his high school newspaper in St. Cloud, Minnesota. He then went to the University of California, Berkeley, where he graduated with honors in linguistics, writing his honors thesis on language acquisition in autistic children.

Today, he lives in Scottsdale, Arizona with his wife Lauren and five daughters. Dr. Loes sees private patients and devotes time to education and research.

REFERENCES

1 A.B. Roberts and M.B. Sporn, eds., "Peptide Growth Factors and Their Receptors: in *The Transforming Growth Factors-ℨ: Handbook of Experimental Pharmacology* (New York: Springer-Verlag, 1990), 419-720.

2 A.B. Roberts and M.B. Sporn, "The Molecular and Cellular Biology of Wound Repair" in *Transforming Growth Factor- ℨ* ; Clark RAF ed., (New York Plenum Press, 1996), 275-308.

3 J.I. Gallin and R. Snyderman, *Inflammation, Basic Principles and Clinical Correlates*, 3rd ed., (Lippincott Williams & Wildins, 1999), IBIN: 0397517599.

4 G.D. Blobe, W.P. Schiemann and H.F. Lodish, "Rose of Transforming Growth Factor ℨ in Human Disease," *New England Journal of Medicine*, *Vol 342, No 18, (April 2000): 1350-1358. NOTE: the next reference in the text is in chapter 7 relating to the Hanes Study. Ferkitch A.K., Schwartzbaum Ph.D., Frid D.J., Moeschberger M.D., Archives of Internal Medicine, 2000:160:1261-1268).

5 (Ferkitch AK., Schwartzbaum Ph.D. Frid DJ., Moeschberger ML, *Archives of Internal Medicine*, 2000:160:1261-1268)

6 M. Pimentel, et al. "Eradication of Small Intestinal Bacterial Overgrowth Reduces Symptoms of Irritable Bowel Syndrome." *American Journal of Gastroenterology*, 2000;95(12):3503.

7 Nobaek, S., et al. "Alteration of intestinal microflora is associated with reduction in abdominal bloating and pain in patients with irritable bowel syndrome." *Am J Gastroenterol*, 2000;95(5):1231-1238.

8 King, T.S., et al. "Abnormal colonic fermentation in irritable bowel syndrome." *Lancet*, 1998;352(9135):1187-1189.

9 Murray, M. *5-HTTP: The Natural Way to Overcome Depression, Obesity, and Insomnia*. New York: Bantam Books, 1999.

10 Titus, F., et al. "5-hydroxytryptophan versus methysergide in the prophylaxis of migraine: randomized clinical trial." *European Neurology*; 1986;25:327-329.

11 Sicuteri, F. "5-hydroxytryptophan in the prophylaxis of migraine." *Pharmacological Research Communications*, 1972;5:213-218.

12 Sicuteri, F. "The ingestion of serotonin precursors (L-5-hydroxytryptophan and L-tryptophan) improves migraine." *Headache*, 1973;13:19-22.

13 De Giorgis, G., et al. "Headache in association with sleep disorders in children: a psychodiagnostic evaluation and controlled clinical study—L-5-HTP versus placebo." *Drugs Under Experimental and Clinical Research*, 1987;13:425-433.

14 Battistella, P.A., et al. "Beta-endorphin in plasma and monocytes in juvenile headache." *Headache*, 1996;36:91-94.